Pocket Book of Ophthalmology

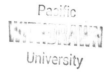

Pocket Book of

Ophthalmology

Philip I. Murray PhD, FRCS, FRCOphth.
Senior Lecturer in Ophthalmology, University of Birmingham,
Birmingham and Midland Eye Centre, Birmingham

Alistair R. Fielder FRCP, FRCS, FRCOphth.
Kennerley Bankes Professor of Ophthalmology, Academic Unit of
Ophthalmology, The Western Eye Hospital, Imperial College School
of Medicine at St. Mary's, London

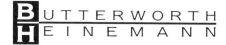

BUTTERWORTH
HEINEMANN

Butterworth-Heinemann
Linacre House, Jordan Hill, Oxford OX2 8DP
A division of Reed Educational and Professional Publishing Ltd

ℛ A member of the Reed Elsevier group

OXFORD BOSTON JOHANNESBURG
MELBOURNE NEW DELHI SINGAPORE

First published 1997

British Library Cataloguing in Publication Data
A catalogue record for this book is available from the British Library

Library of Congress Cataloguing in Publication Data
A catalogue record for this book is available from the Library of Congress

ISBN 0 7506 2371 3

Composition by Scribe Design, Gillingham, Kent
Printed and bound in Great Britain by Hartnolls Ltd, Bodmin, Cornwall

Contents

A. Introduction vii

B. Applied anatomy and physiology 1

C. Conditions 11

Acute anterior uveitis 11

Age-related macular degeneration 12

Alkali burns 13

Anterior ischaemic optic neuropathy 14

Basal cell carcinoma 15

Blepharitis 15

Cataract 16

Conjunctivitis – bacterial 18

Conjunctivitis – viral 19

Corneal abrasion 19

Corneal foreign body 20

Cytomegalovirus retinitis 21

Demyelinating disease 23

Diabetic retinopathy 24

Dry eye 25

Dysthyroid ophthalmopathy 26

Ectropion 28

Entropion 28

Episcleritis 29

Eye movement disorders 30

Giant cell arteritis 31

Glaucoma 33

Glaucoma – infantile 35

Hypertensive retinopathy 36

Keratitis – bacterial 37

Keratitis – marginal 38

Keratitis – viral 39

Keratoconus 40

Leukocoria 41

Malignant melanoma 42

Meibomian cyst 43

Nystagmus 44

Optic atrophy 45

Papilloedema 46

Posterior vitreous detachment 47

Ptosis 48

Pupil responses – abnormal 50

Retinal artery occlusion 51

Contents

Retinal detachment 52
Retinal vein occlusion 53
Retinitis pigmentosa 54
Retinoblastoma 55
Retinopathy of prematurity 56
Sarcoidosis 58
Scleritis 59
Sickle cell retinopathy 60
Strabismus (squint) 61
Toxoplasmosis 64
Trauma 66
Vernal keratoconjunctivitis 68
The watery eye 69

D. Topics 71
Assessment 71
History taking 71
Common symptomatology 72
Differential diagnosis of red eye 73
Painless loss of vision 76
Painful loss of vision 76
Visual fields 76
Fluorescein angiography 78
Ultrasonography and biometry 79
Electrophysiology 80
Ageing and the visual system 82
Eye as a clue to metabolic disease 83
Genetics in ophthalmology 84
Common ophthalmological instruments 86
Vision and optics 89
Visual acuity 89
Near acuity 90
Refractive error 90
Accommodation 93
Spectacles 94
Contact lenses 95
Visual acuity testing in children 96
Therapeutic 99
Ocular pharmacology 99
Lasers 100
E. Appendix – useful diagrams 103
Index 107

The purpose of this book is to provide an outline of common ophthalmological conditions and to encourage an interest in the specialty. It is not a comprehensive textbook or a book of lists but should be used as a guide to ophthalmology and as an adjunct to wider reading. It has been devised to fit into a pocket and would be readily at hand to give a brief overview and understanding of ophthalmological disease encountered in an eye clinic and in general practice. Although aimed at undergraduates and general practitioners, the book would be of value to physicians with an interest in ophthalmology, optometrists, orthoptists, ophthalmic nurses and visual field technicians.

Philip I. Murray
Alistair R. Fielder

The visual system consists of a coordinated pair of eyes, the appropriate protective mechanisms and the necessary neural apparatus to interpret visual information. The anterior visual pathway consists of the retina, optic nerve, chiasm and optic tracts. The posterior visual pathway consists of the lateral geniculate nucleus (LGN), optic radiations, visual cortex and visual association areas. The total power of the eye is 58 dioptres with the cornea being the most powerful refracting surface of the eye (48 dioptres), yet to form an image on the retina an additional adjustable focusing element, the crystalline lens is needed.

Requirements
- Formation of a focused image on the retina depends on:
  - Ocular shape, resulting from its mechanical properties and the intraocular pressure
  - Transparency of the ocular media
  - Ability of transparent structures to refract light
- Transduction and interpretation of the image
  - The retina converts light energy into nervous impulses – a process termed transduction. The path connecting the retinal photoreceptor to the visual cortex has three neurons: 1) the bipolar cell, 2) the ganglion cell, both located in the retina; and 3) a final neuron with its cell body in the LGN which projects to the cerebral cortex
- The integration of visual information from both eyes

Cornea
- Transparent, avascular tissue
- Forms approximately the anterior 1/6 of the outer coat of the eye and is continuous posteriorly with the sclera
- Has five layers comprising:
  - epithelium – non-keratinized, five to seven cells thick, capable of rapid division
  - Bowman's membrane

- Stroma – 90% corneal thickness, glyco-saminoglycan matrix, collagen fibrils
- Descemet's membrane
- Endothelium – single layer of non-regenerating cells
◆ Functions include:
  - Transparency
    * The state of relative dehydration of the stroma is maintained by both the impermeable epithelial barrier and active pumping mechanisms of the corneal endothelium
    * The regular spacing of individual stromal collagen fibrils
  - Refraction – the cornea is the major refractive component of the eye
  - Barrier to infection and trauma

Sclera
◆ Opaque, mechanically tough
◆ Forms the posterior 5/6 of the outer coat of the eye
◆ Consists of irregularly arranged collagen fibres
◆ Functions include:
  - Maintenance of the constancy of ocular shape
  - Maintenance of intraocular pressure
  - Barrier to infection and trauma

Aqueous humour
◆ Constituents essentially similar to plasma but only 1% of the plasma protein concentration, and a high ascorbic acid level
◆ Functions are to:
  - Maintain intraocular pressure
  - Contribute to ocular transparency
  - Provide metabolic support for the lens, cornea and vitreous
◆ Aqueous formation:
  - Active secretion by the epithelium of the ciliary body (major component)

- Passive diffusion in the region of the ciliary body (minor component)
◆ Aqueous drainage:
    - Passes through the pupil and drains out of the eye mainly by pressure dependent flow, through the angle of the anterior chamber through the sieve-like trabecular meshwork. Aqueous reaches the canal of Schlemm, a modified vein, and then enters the vascular system on the surface of the sclera

Intraocular pressure (IOP)
◆ IOP is maintained at its normal level of 10-21 mmHg by the dynamic balance between secretion and drainage of aqueous humour

Crystalline lens
◆ A biconvex structure with an outer acellular capsule
◆ Consists of very tightly packed hexagonal fibres
◆ The cortex contains the more recently formed fibres
◆ The nucleus contains the older, non-dividing cells
◆ Has a relatively low water (66%) and high protein (35%) content (crystallins)
◆ Functions:
    - Transparency, due to:
        * Orderly arrangement of the lens fibres
        * Small difference in refractive index between the various components
        * Absence of blood vessels
◆ Focusing
◆ A range of congenital, age-related, or metabolic (e.g. diabetic) changes in the lens fibres lead to structural irregularity with resultant opacification, i.e. cataract formation

Vitreous
◆ Firm gel with a volume of 4 ml occupying 80% of the globe volume

◆ Composition:
 – Major structural protein is collagen type II, arranged in fibrils
 – Contains only a few cells (hyalocytes), which secrete the glycosaminoglycan hyaluronic acid which fills the spaces between the collagen lamellae
◆ Functions are to:
 – Maintain transparency
 – Protect the ocular structures by mechanical buffering
 – Passive 'transport and removal' of metabolites

Retina
◆ Complex structure (containing 120 million rods and 6 million cones) of many layers but can be simplified considerably to:
 – Four layers of cells
   * The retinal pigment epithelium (RPE)
   * Photoreceptors (rods and cones)
   * Intermediary cells which comprise: Bipolar, amacrine, horizontal and Müller cells
   * Ganglion cells
 – Two interconnecting layers – inner and outer plexiform layers
 – Two membranes – inner and outer limiting membranes
◆ Is transparent because of its
 – Thinness
 – Relative absence of blood vessels (especially in the foveal region)
 – The regular, columnar arrangement of its cells
◆ Macular region – diameter 5.5 mm, lies lateral (3.5 mm) and slightly inferior (1.0 mm) to the optic disc. This area is cone-rich, ophthalmoscopically ill-defined and slightly darker than

the rest of the retina due partly to the accumulation of yellow luteal pigment. The macula is subdivided into:

- Fovea – diameter 1.9 mm – area is rod-free and devoid of ganglion cells
- Foveola – diameter 0.35 mm – a pit in the centre of the fovea and also rod-free, has cones in their greatest density – hence the high visual acuity from this area, and is capillary-free, as blood vessels would interfere with vision

Optic nerve

◆ Containing just over 1 million fibres of second order neurons, with their cell bodies in the ganglion cells of the retina and terminating in the LGN

◆ Nerve fibres are myelinated only after leaving the eye – there is no myelination of nerve fibres in the retina, as this would impede vision

◆ Optic disc
  - the entry of the optic nerve into the eye (1.5 × 1.5 mm) and corresponds to the blind spot of the visual field, as it does not contain any overlying retinal photoreceptors

Optic chiasm

◆ Major feature is that about 50% optic nerve fibres decussate here. Thus fibres from the nasal retina cross to enter the opposite optic tract while those from the temporal retina enter the ipsilateral optic tract

◆ Fibres in the inferonasal chiasm enter the opposite optic nerve for a short way before passing back to enter the corresponding optic tract. This loop is an important localizing diagnostic aid, as a compressive pituitary lesion at this site leads to a characteristic visual field defect

Optic tract
◆ Extends from the optic chiasm to the LGN
◆ Contains uncrossed and crossed fibres from the temporal and nasal retinas, respectively
◆ About 30% fibres leave the visual pathway in the optic tract, before the LGN, including those subserving the pupillary light reflex, which pass to the pretectal nuclei – this is important clinically and explains why the pupillary reflex remains intact in lesions of the visual cortex

Lateral geniculate nucleus
◆ Part of the thalamus, has six laminae and contains the nuclei for the third neuron of the visual pathway
◆ There is accurate point-to-point representation of the retina
◆ The LGN laminae keep information from each eye separate

Optic radiations
◆ Axons of the third neuron of the visual pathway originate in the LGN
◆ The anteroinferior radiation fans out as Meyer's loop by passing down into the temporal lobe. A lesion of Meyer's loop causes an upper homonymous temporal 'pie-in-the-sky' visual field defect

Visual cortex
◆ The primary visual cortex (Brodman's area 17) lies in the interhemispheric fissure and extends posteriorly about 1–2 cm onto the posterior surface of the cortex
◆ The visual cortex lies on either side of the calcarine fissure for about 5 cm and extends further anteriorly along the inferior border
◆ Only in the cortex is there integration of inputs from both eyes allowing binocular vision

Visual association areas
◆ For detailed and higher interpretation, information must be passed to other cortical areas; these include Brodman's areas 18 and 19, also known as the parastriate and peristriate areas

Arrangement of fibres in the visual pathway – overview
◆ The inferior retina is projected into the superior visual field – there is an inverted relationship between the visual system and the visual field
◆ Fibres are rearranged along the visual pathway. Thus moving back towards the chiasm the macular fibres serving central vision tend to be arranged in the centre of the nerve
◆ Fibres from the nasal retina decussate into the opposite optic tract at the chiasm
◆ Lesions posterior to the chiasm produce homonymous visual field defects which are more congruous, the more posterior the lesion
◆ There is accurate point-to-point (retinotopic) representation in the posterior visual pathway (LGN and cortex)

Visual processing
Once an image is formed on the retina, transduction of light energy into neural information is performed by the retinal photoreceptors. The physiological processes of vision can be divided into:
◆ Light sense
  – The ability to detect the presence and intensity of light (visible spectrum 400–760 nm)
  – The chemical changes affecting the photoreceptors on exposure to light
  – Daylight is optimum for cone vision (photopic vision)
  – With reducing illumination, vision becomes rod dependent (scotopic vision)

◆ Colour sense
 – Four pigment types are known:
   * Rhodopsin in rods
   * Short, medium, and long wavelength iodopsins, three pigments in cones which are sensitive to blue, green and red light, respectively
◆ Form sense
 – The ability to discriminate and interpret different parts of the visual image by the analysis of its contours and contrast; this includes:
   * Visual acuity, i.e. the ability to see fine detail
   * Contrast sensitivity, i.e. the 'real-life' dimension of the amount of contrast which exists between the object of interest and its surroundings

Integration of visual information from both eyes
◆ The mechanisms which enable the two eyes to move and work as a single functional unit include:
 – Extraocular muscles
 – Control of eye movements
   * Infranuclear pathways – course of the III, IV, VI cranial nerves. Infranuclear lesions only affect the movement of one eye
   * Cranial nerve nuclei and the supranuclear pathways. The supranuclear pathways (e.g. the medial longitudinal fasciculus of the brainstem) connect the various cranial nerve nuclei, and also relay impulses from the various parts of the cortex (e.g. frontomesencephalic), cerebellum, brainstem, and neck
 – Binocular vision
   * The presence of a pair of eyes whose function as a unit is greater than the sum of the function of each individual eye

(binocular summation), this allows a greater visual field and, by overlapping the fields, perception of depth by stereopsis. The prerequisites for binocular vision are:

* Both eyes must act in concert
* Good vision is required from each eye
* The line of sight of each eye must at all times be pointing towards the same visual target

ACUTE ANTERIOR UVEITIS

Inflammation of the iris (iritis, acute iridocyclitis). UVEITIS CANNOT BE ACCURATELY DIAGNOSED WITHOUT SLIT-LAMP EXAMINATION, SO REFER TO AN EYE UNIT

Causes
◆ majority unknown, occurs usually in 20–50 year age group
◆ as 50% are HLA B27 +ve there is an association with ankylosing spondylitis

Symptoms
◆ red eye (usually unilateral)
◆ pain
◆ blurred vision
◆ photophobia
◆ (may be history of previous attack)

Examination
◆ conjunctival injection (circumcorneal injection, ciliary flush)
◆ keratic precipitates (inflammatory cells) on corneal endothelium
◆ flare (albumin leakage from iris vessels) and (inflammatory) cells in the anterior chamber, hypopyon if severe
◆ miosis and posterior synechiae (adhesions between iris and lens, PS)

Complications
◆ may be associated with raised intraocular pressure (IOP)
◆ 360° PS formation leads to blockage of aqueous humour circulation leading to iris bombé and high IOP
◆ may become chronic and develop secondary cataract ± macular oedema leading to reduced vision
◆ the condition is likely to recur and in either eye

Treatment
- dilate pupil to prevent ciliary spasm and break posterior synechiae
- intensive topical steroids (drops), initially 1–2 hourly then gradually reduce over next 4–6 weeks
- in severe cases a subconjunctival injection of steroid ± mydricaine (dilating agent) is necessary

AGE-RELATED MACULAR DEGENERATION

Age related disease involving the macula, usually bilateral. In developed countries commonest causes of blindness over the age of 65

Cause
- unknown

Symptoms
- gradual or sudden loss of central vision with difficulty reading
- usually slow progression (years)
- distortion often first symptom
- eventually severe loss of central field but maintain peripheral navigational vision
- if associated with haemorrhage may have sudden deterioration

Examination
- drusen: white/yellow spots at the macula
- atrophic changes with loss of foveal reflex and increased pigmentation at posterior pole
- retinal oedema and haemorrhage at the posterior pole (disciform – subretinal neovascular membrane)

Treatment
- low vision aids (magnifiers) to help reading
- some with disciform may respond to laser treatment in very early stages only
- blind/partial sight registration

Complications
- leading cause of registerable blindness in the elderly
- patients will not go completely 'blind'; they keep their independence as peripheral vision is maintained

ALKALI BURNS

Severe, destructive chemical burn that may result in permanent visual loss. Usually occurs from assault with an ammonia solution, or accidentally from cement particles in building workers

Symptoms
- pain
- burning
- loss of vision
- redness

Examination
- may be reduced visual acuity
- red eye(s)
- corneal epithelial loss (may be total loss)
- corneal clouding
- conjunctival epithelial loss
- ischaemia of corneal limbus (the more the ischaemia, the worse the prognosis)
- anterior uveitis
- raised intraocular pressure
- cataract

Complications
- failure of cornea to re-epithelialize
- secondary bacterial keratitis
- corneal opacification
- corneal neovascularization
- corneal perforation
- conjunctival scarring and shrinkage

Treatment
- IMMEDIATE copious irrigation with water
- removal of cement particles
- admit if moderate/severe damage
- topical antibiotic (to prevent secondary infection)
- topical dilation (to help pain)
- topical and oral vitamin C (to aid collagen synthesis)
- topical steroids (to reduce inflammation)
- conjunctival/corneal grafting may be required

ANTERIOR ISCHAEMIC OPTIC NEUROPATHY

Occlusion of the short posterior ciliary arteries which supply the optic nerve head. Usually in middle aged/elderly patients

Causes
- non-arteritic (arteriosclerosis/atherosclerosis)
- arteritic (giant cell arteritis)

Symptoms
- painless, sudden loss of vision

Examination
- gross reduction in visual acuity
- relative afferent pupillary defect
- pale, swollen optic disc with surrounding nerve fibre haemorrhages
- disc swelling may be segmental, often affecting superior part of disc with corresponding inferior altitudinal field defect

Complications
- blindness
- optic atrophy
- unusual for fellow eye to be involved if non-arteritic

Treatment
- if arteritic (see GIANT CELL ARTERITIS)
- if non-arteritic, treat underlying medical condition, e.g. hypertension

BASAL CELL CARCINOMA

Commonest malignant eyelid tumour, also known as a rodent ulcer

Symptoms
- 'lump' on eyelid slowly increasing in size
- occasionally 'lump' may bleed

Examination
- lesion usually lower lid or medial canthus
- classically pearly margin with blood vessels and a central shallow ulcerated base
- occasionally less clearly defined margins (morphoeic type)

Complications
- spread by direct extension with invasion of local structures
- does not metastasize
- may recur if not completely excised

Treatment
- surgery
- radiotherapy
- cryotherapy

BLEPHARITIS

Chronic inflammation of the eyelid margins

Causes
- usually *Staphylococcus aureus* or *epidermidis*
- associated with skin disease, e.g. acne rosacea, seborrhoeic dermatitis

Symptoms
- sore, gritty, occasionally red eyes

Examination
- hyperaemic lid margins
- crusts on lashes
- blocked meibomian gland orifices
- meibomian cysts

Complications
- conjunctivitis
- marginal keratitis
- meibomian cysts

Treatment
- lid hygiene with sodium bicarbonate
- lubricants
- antibiotic ointment
- low-dose systemic (oxy)tetracycline

CATARACT

Opacification of the natural lens – commonest types are nuclear sclerosis (yellow/brown lens, may cause acquired myopia), cortical, and posterior subcapsular (causes glare; this type may also be associated with intraocular inflammation and systemic steroid use)

Causes
- ageing (commonest, almost everybody >65 years has some degree of cataract)
- secondary to ocular disease (e.g. glaucoma, intraocular inflammation)
- secondary to systemic disease (e.g. rubella, diabetes mellitus, myotonic dystrophy)
- congenital

Symptoms
- gradual blurred vision
- glare

Examination
- grey/white pupil using a pen torch
- reduced red reflex

Treatment
In the absence of effective medical treatment, surgery is the only option although early on spectacles often help

Cataract surgery
Indicated when the level of vision restricts normal activity
◆ most commonly performed intraocular operation,
◆ usually results in excellent return of vision if no other ocular pathology present

Phacoemulsification and posterior chamber intraocular lens (IOL) implant
◆ increasingly popular
◆ mainly LA (day case) or GA
◆ small incision
◆ removal of anterior lens capsule
◆ high speed vibrating tip cuts nucleus into tiny particles and aspirates them
◆ irrigation and aspiration of remaining cortex
◆ retains posterior capsule
◆ insertion of foldable (e.g. silicone) posterior chamber IOL into capsular bag
◆ no sutures – reduced astigmatism
◆ fast healing and visual rehabilitation

Extracapsular cataract extraction and posterior chamber intraocular lens (IOL) implant

Procedure
◆ until recently most common procedure
◆ incision in superior part of cornea or at the corneoscleral junction
◆ removal of anterior lens capsule
◆ manual expression of lens nucleus
◆ irrigation and aspiration of remaining cortex
◆ retains posterior capsule
◆ insertion of posterior chamber (PMMA) IOL into capsular bag
◆ suturing of wound (10/0 nylon)

- larger incision
- slower healing and visual rehabilitation

Complications
- per-operative (rupture of the posterior capsule, vitreous loss – anterior chamber lens implant inserted)
- post-operative – uveitis, glaucoma, retinal detachment, endophthalmitis (all infrequent)
- astigmatism (sutures too tight but they can be easily removed at the slit lamp)

Postoperative treatment
- topical steroids
- topical antibiotics
- pupil mobility (topical mydriatic)

CONJUNCTIVITIS – BACTERIAL

Bacterial infection of the conjunctiva

Causes
- usually *Staphylococcus, streptococcus* or *Haemophilus* species

Symptoms
- slight discomfort
- red, sticky eye(s)
- visual acuity is not affected although slight blurring due to purulent exudation, which clears when discharge is blinked away

Examination
- generalized conjunctival injection with purulent discharge
- lashes may stick together
- both eyes may be involved

Complications
- usually nil

Treatment
- topical antibiotic (e.g. fusidic acid bd, chloramphenicol – hourly for 24 h then qid for a week)
- general hygiene by not sharing towels etc.

CONJUNCTIVITIS – VIRAL

Viral infection of the conjunctiva

Causes
- usually adenovirus (self-limiting, but can also affect cornea – keratoconjunctivitis)

Symptoms
- red, watery eye(s)
- gritty, uncomfortable feeling

Examination
- generalized conjunctival injection with watery discharge
- follicles (lymphoid aggregates) in the tarsal conjunctiva
- enlarged pre-auricular lymph node
- petechial conjunctival haemorrhages
- both eyes may be involved
- associated upper respiratory tract infection

Complications
- highly contagious
- may last several weeks
- small corneal opacities leading to photophobia and reduced vision

Treatment
- nil
- antibiotic drops (e.g. chloramphenicol) qid to prevent secondary bacterial infection
- general hygiene by not sharing towels etc.

CORNEAL ABRASION

Loss of corneal epithelium

Causes
◆ trauma, e.g. foreign object, child's fingernail

Symptoms
◆ red, watery eye
◆ moderate to severe pain
◆ blurred vision
◆ photophobia

Examination
◆ conjunctival injection
◆ loss of epithelium stains green with fluorescein drops using a 'blue' torch
◆ linear scratches are usually secondary to a sub-tarsal FB
◆ miosis usually when there is marked photophobia

Complications
◆ occasionally leads to bacterial keratitis
◆ recurrent abrasion (erosion) where the epithelium repeatedly breaks down in an area where there has been a previous abrasion

Treatment
◆ dilate pupil to prevent ciliary spasm, antibiotic drop/ointment, pad eye
◆ may need a few days of padding before epithelium heals
◆ then antibiotic drops/ointment for 1 week to prevent secondary bacterial infection and to keep the cornea lubricated

CORNEAL FOREIGN BODY

Foreign material embedded in corneal epithelium/stroma

Causes
- metal or vegetable
- industrial environment (failure to wear goggles if grinding)
- domestic (gardening, farming)
- chance, e.g. windy day

Symptoms
- red, watery eye
- foreign body (FB) feeling

Examination
- conjunctival injection
- small FB on cornea (if metal, may have surrounding rust ring)

Complications
- very occasionally leads to bacterial keratitis
- suspect penetration of the globe if no FB is seen especially after drilling with power tools, even if minor/no symptoms and normal vision – X-RAY TO EXCLUDE A RADIO-OPAQUE INTRAOCULAR FB

Treatment
- instil topical local anaesthetic and remove FB (± rust ring) with cotton wool bud, needle tip or small rotary drill
- instil topical antibiotic and pad eye (may need rust ring removing the following day as it can prevent healing)
- topical antibiotic qid for 1 week to prevent secondary bacterial infection

CYTOMEGALOVIRUS RETINITIS

Cytomegalovirus (CMV) is a member of the herpes group of DNA viruses. CMV retinitis is the commonest AIDS-related opportunistic infection of the eye. It occurs in about 25% of AIDS patients and those with an absolute CD4+ level of <50 cells/mm^3 are at greatest risk of developing the disease.

Symptoms
- may be minimal
- photopsia (flashes)
- visual field loss
- reduced visual acuity

Clinical Findings
- slowly, progressive necrotizing retinitis, unilateral or bilateral
- white intraretinal lesions and areas of infiltrate and necrosis are associated with prominent retinal haemorrhage ('pizza pie' appearance)
- peripherally, it has a less intense white appearance with areas of granular, white retinitis that may or may not have associated haemorrhage ('brush fire' appearance)
- minimal vitreous activity

Treatment
- 14 day induction course of i.v. ganciclovir or foscarnet
- lifelong maintenance therapy required and indwelling central venous catheter inserted
- 80–100% initial response to therapy with either drug but up to 50% of patients will get a recurrence within 3 months and in most cases a reinduction course will be effective
- if treatment is stopped, active retinitis recurs in virtually all patients within 3–4 weeks
- ganciclovir also available as oral, intravitreal preparations and as an intraocular device
- i.v. cidofovir now available

Complications
- related to the ocular disease and/or treatment
- blindness may result from retinal detachment (in 30% of patients) or optic nerve head involvement
- a long-term indwelling central venous line exposes the patient to the risk of catheter-related infection, sepsis or thrombosis

- ◆ ganciclovir may cause neutropenia
- ◆ foscarnet may cause renal toxicity
- ◆ CMV retinitis may also co-exist with other opportunistic infections

DEMYELINATING DISEASE

Ocular manifestations of multiple sclerosis (MS)

Optic neuritis

Symptoms
- ◆ sudden/recent loss of central vision
- ◆ worse on exercise or having a bath (Uhthoff's phenomenon)
- ◆ pain on ocular movement
- ◆ colour desaturation

Examination
- ◆ reduced visual acuity
- ◆ central or paracentral scotoma
- ◆ diminished red/green colour vision
- ◆ relative afferent pupillary defect
- ◆ normal optic disc (retrobulbar neuritis)
- ◆ swollen optic disc (papillitis)
- ◆ abnormal visual evoked response

Natural history
- ◆ usually visual acuity returns almost to normal after 6 weeks but permanent visual loss can occur
- ◆ temporal pallor of optic disc
- ◆ MS may occur in up to 75% of patients

Treatment
- ◆ usually nil
- ◆ systemic corticosteroids will hasten the resolution but the final visual outcome is not affected
- ◆ intravenous methylprednisolone may protect against the onset of MS

Internuclear ophthalmoplegia
Results from a lesion in the medial longitudinal fasciculus

Symptoms
◆ do not usually complain of double vision

Examination
◆ limitation of adduction of one eye
◆ nystagmus of the fellow eye on abduction
◆ usually bilateral in MS (unilateral in arterio-sclerosis)
◆ normal convergence

DIABETIC RETINOPATHY

Microvascular disease of the retinal microcirculation
◆ COMMONEST CAUSE OF BLINDNESS UNDER 65 YEARS
◆ strict diabetic control may partially protect against retinopathy

Symptoms
◆ usually none until:
  – gradual loss of vision – central (macular area) retina is involved by oedema, exudation or haemorrhage
  – sudden loss of vision – most commonly vitreous haemorrhage

Maculopathy
◆ involves predominantly the central retinal region

Symptoms
◆ distortion of central vision with difficulty reading

Examination
◆ oedema, exudates, microaneurysms and haemorrhages at macula

Treatment
◆ some respond well to focal laser photocoagulation

Retinopathy

Stage	Examination	Treatment
Background	microaneurysms, haemorrhages, exudates	observe or laser photocoagulation depending if central vision threatened
Preproliferative	cotton wool spots, venous beading, looping of vessels	careful observation by ophthalmologist
Proliferative (more common in type 1 diabetes)	fine new vessels on disc or elsewhere ± vitreous haemorrhage	urgent panretinal laser photocoagulation
End Stage	fibrosis, tractional retinal detachment	vitreoretinal surgery

DRY EYE

Failure of the tear film to wet the ocular surface

Causes
◆ decreased tear secretion
 – keratoconjunctivitis sicca
  * associated with rheumatoid arthritis
  * Sjögren's syndrome (also dry mouth – xerostomia)
 – cicatricial conjunctivitis
  * trachoma
  * chemical burns
  * pemphigoid
  * erythema multiforme (Stevens–Johnson syndrome)
 – trigeminal nerve defect
 – facial nerve defect
◆ tear film abnormalities
 – blepharitis (meibomian gland dysfunction)

Symptoms
- burning
- FB feeling
- redness

Examination
- decreased pre-corneal tear film
- decreased Schirmer test (strip of filter paper placed in inferior conjunctival fornix and the length of paper wetted over a 4-min period is measured – normal is 10–25 mm)
- corneal/conjunctival staining after instillation of the dye Rose Bengal (the dryer the eye the more uncomfortable are the drops)
- filaments of mucus on cornea
- corneal/conjunctival scarring if cicatricial disease
- with blepharitis may also have a watery eye (tears are the wrong consistency – too oily – and do not stay on the eye long enough to wet the eye so they overflow down the cheek)

Complications
- of decreased tear secretion
  - keratinization of corneal and conjunctival epithelium
  - secondary bacterial keratitis
  - corneal perforation

Treatment
- frequent artificial tear substitutes
- topical mucolytic, e.g. acetylcysteine
- topical antibiotic to prevent secondary infection
- occlusion of lower lacrimal puncta
- lid hygiene with sodium bicarbonate for blepharitis

DYSTHYROID OPHTHALMOPATHY

Eye and orbital changes usually seen in association with thyroid gland dysfunction. Occasionally patient is clinically and biochemically euthyroid

Causes
- probable immunologically mediated disease

Symptoms
- nil
- grittiness
- redness
- lid swelling
- double vision
- unsightly cosmetic appearance, 'bulgy' eye(s)
- visual loss

Examination
- signs may be unilateral or bilateral
- injection over insertion of rectus muscles especially medial rectus
- lid oedema
- lid lag
- upper and lower lid retraction
- proptosis (exophthalmos)
- diplopia due to reduced ocular motility, especially upgaze and abduction due to enlargement of medial and inferior recti
- corneal exposure with ulceration in severe cases
- optic nerve compression with reduced vision, relative afferent pupil defect, field loss, reduced colour vision
- gross enlargement of extraocular muscles seen on CT scan
- abnormal thyroid function tests (usually hyperthyroid)

Complications
- blindness due to:
  - optic nerve compression
  - corneal perforation
- cosmetic disfigurement

Treatment
- nil
- manage thyroid dysfunction

◆ ocular lubricants
◆ for optic nerve compression:
  – surgical orbital decompression
  – systemic corticosteroids
  – radiotherapy
◆ lid and extraocular muscle surgery once the active phase is over (usually 12–18 months)
◆ prisms on spectacles for diplopia
◆ botulinum toxin injection for diplopia

ECTROPION

Eversion of the lower lid

Causes
◆ ageing (commonest)
◆ VII cranial nerve palsy
◆ cicatricial

Symptoms
◆ watery eye

Examination
◆ everted lower lid easily seen with naked eye
◆ may be small medial ectropion only

Complications
◆ exposed eye leading to drying of the conjunctiva

Treatment
◆ lubrication to prevent drying due to exposure
◆ long-term correction with surgical procedure under LA

ENTROPION

An inturning of the lid, usually the lower

Causes
◆ ageing (commonest)

◆ cicatricial, e.g. following trachoma infection in the tropics

Symptoms
◆ irritation, foreign body feeling

Examination
◆ if not present, ask patient to close eyes tightly – then open

Complications
◆ eyelashes rubbing on cornea leading to keratitis and reduced vision

Treatment
◆ topical antibiotic to prevent infection
◆ taping down the lower lid (temporary measure)
◆ long-term correction with surgical procedure under LA

EPISCLERITIS

Benign inflammation of the fibroelastic tissue covering the sclera

Causes
◆ usually unknown
◆ occasionally associated with systemic disease, e.g. rheumatological disorder

Symptoms
◆ red eye(s)
◆ mild discomfort/ache

Examination
◆ diffuse or nodular areas of hyperaemia in one or both eyes
◆ normal visual acuity

Complications
◆ usually nil

Treatment
- ◆ may be self-limiting so no treatment is required
- ◆ oral NSAID, e.g flurbiprofen 50–100 mg tds
- ◆ topical steroids

EYE MOVEMENT DISORDERS

Eye movement disorders are very difficult to classify, being relatively infrequent; only certain aspects are included here.

Nuclear and infranuclear disorders
Affect the movement of ONE eye only, unless the lesion is bilateral
  The site of the lesion can be in the cranial nerve nucleus, or anywhere along the peripheral nerve: in the brainstem, cavernous sinus, orbit, or muscle
If only one function of a multifunction cranial nerve is involved (e.g. III) the lesion is either in the brainstem or orbit

Causes
- ◆ **cranial nerve lesions of III, IV or VI**
  - – vascular occlusive disease as a mini-stroke
  - – compressive by tumour or aneurysm etc.
  - – inflammatory, e.g. in orbit or cavernous sinus
  - – following neurosurgery
- ◆ **muscle disease**
  - – myasthenia gravis
  - – there are others but very rare

Symptoms
- ◆ diplopia – binocular diplopia, due to misalignment of the eyes, must be differentiated
  from monocular, due to cataract etc., the former disappears when one eye is closed, the latter persists when using each eye individually
- ◆ other symptoms depend on cause of nerve palsy or muscle disease

Examination
◆ ocular movements
◆ full neurological examination

The aim of assessment is to distinguish between a serious, neurological disorder requiring very urgent action, from an ophthalmic disorder, which although important is not in itself life-threatening

Treatment
◆ the underlying cause
◆ diplopia
  – patch eye – temporary only
  – prisms
  – botulinum toxin
  – strabismus surgery

Supranuclear disorders
Affect the movements of BOTH eyes as the lesion is central to the cranial nerve nucleus. Such disorders include gaze and internuclear palsies and are encountered in demyelinating conditions, cerebral: tumours, haemorrhage, infarct etc.

GIANT CELL ARTERITIS

Systemic vasculitis affecting arteries. Usually occurs >60 years and is commoner in females

Symptoms
◆ temporal headache
◆ pain on chewing
◆ general malaise
◆ loss of appetite
◆ loss of weight
◆ pain on brushing hair (scalp tenderness)
◆ girdle pain/stiffness/weakness (associated with polymyalgia rheumatica)

♦ transient loss of vision in one eye (amaurosis fugax)
♦ sudden loss of vision
♦ diplopia

Examination
♦ tenderness of superficial temporal arteries
♦ anterior ischaemic optic neuropathy with swollen optic disc and altitudinal field defect and gross reduction of visual acuity
♦ VI cranial nerve palsy
♦ occasionally central retinal artery occlusion

Diagnosis
♦ characteristic history (symptoms)
♦ raised ESR
♦ raised C-reactive protein
♦ superficial temporal artery biopsy
    - for the definitive diagnosis
    - histology shows artery wall thickened by inflammatory infiltrate including giant cells
    - should be performed within 48 h of starting steroid therapy

Complications
♦ blindness
♦ if treatment is not started immediately then the fellow eye may be involved or a cerebro-vascular accident could occur

Treatment
♦ TREAT AS OPHTHALMIC EMERGENCY TO AVOID BILATERAL BLINDNESS
♦ immediate bolus of intravenous corticosteroid, e.g hydrocortisone (250 mg)/dexamethasone (10 mg) then high dose oral prednisolone (80 mg/day)
♦ taper oral steroids according to ESR and symptoms
♦ long-term oral steroids required

GLAUCOMA

A group of eye conditions characterized by optic disc cupping and visual field loss, in which the intraocular pressure is sufficiently raised to impair normal optic nerve function. Both open angle and acute angle closure glaucoma are rare in young people (<40 years)

Chronic open angle glaucoma
Usually slowly progressive, painless visual loss. Also known as chronic simple glaucoma, primary open angle glaucoma

Causes
- ◆ ageing (increasing incidence with increasing age)
- ◆ steroids (both topical and systemic)
- ◆ inherited (dominant)

Associations
- ◆ family history
- ◆ ocular (high myopia, retinal vein occlusion)
- ◆ systemic (diabetes mellitus)

Symptoms
- ◆ usually none
- ◆ visual loss when condition advanced

Examination/diagnosis
- ◆ reduced visual acuity (advanced disease)
- ◆ raised intraocular pressure >21 mmHg (tonometry)
- ◆ open drainage angle (gonioscopy)
- ◆ pathologically cupped optic discs (cup:disc (C:D) ratio >0.5, pallor, nasal shift of vessels, haemorrhages, asymmetry of C:D ratio)
- ◆ glaucomatous visual field loss

Complications
- ◆ blind eye(s)
- ◆ central retinal vein occlusion

Treatment
Initially medical then surgery for failure of medical treatment

◆ **topical ocular hypotensives**
  - β blockers, e.g. timolol, carteolol, betaxalol, levobunolol
  - sympathomimetics, e.g. adrenaline, dipivefrine
  - parasympathomimetics, e.g. pilocarpine
  - carbonic anhydrase inhibitor, e.g. dorzolamide
  - prostaglandin $F_{2\alpha}$ analogue, e.g. latanoprost
  - α_2 agonists
◆ **systemic hypotensives**
  - carbonic anhydrase inhibitor (acetazolamide), not for long-term therapy
◆ **drainage surgery**
  - trabeculectomy

Acute angle closure glaucoma
Usually sudden (hours), painful visual loss

Causes
◆ primary: hypermetropia (commonest)
◆ secondary: hypermature (swollen) cataract

Symptoms
◆ haloes around lights (when intraocular pressure raised)
◆ reduced vision
◆ ocular pain
◆ headache
◆ nausea and vomiting

Examination
◆ reduced vision
◆ red eye(s)
◆ corneal oedema
◆ mid-dilated, oval pupil
◆ closed drainage angle (gonioscopy)

Complications
◆ blind eye(s)

Treatment
- ◆ initially medical to lower intraocular pressure then laser or surgery is required to allow aquoeus outflow
- ◆ systemic ocular hypotensives
  - – acetazolamide oral/iv
  - – glycerol oral
  - – mannitol i.v.
- ◆ topical
  - – intensive pilocarpine drops
- ◆ YAG laser iridotomy or surgical peripheral iridectomy
  - – laser/surgery is also performed on the unaffected eye to prevent an attack occurring at a later date (prophylaxis)

GLAUCOMA – INFANTILE

A rare, potentially blinding condition which may present at birth or any time in the first 6 months after birth. Characterized by raised intraocular pressure (see section on GLAUCOMA) which may affect one or both eyes. In early infancy, but not later, high intraocular pressure causes the eyeball to enlarge – hence the old term for this type of glaucoma, buphthalmos (ox eye).

Causes
- ◆ developmental abnormality of the drainage mechanism for aqueous humour, probably due to a neural crest abnormality
- ◆ inherited on a multifactorial basis, so boys more frequently affected

Associations
- ◆ may be associated with a wide range of ocular malformations and systemic syndromes

Symptoms
- ◆ photosensitivity – in infancy this is always an important symptom

Examination/diagnosis
- red eye, especially close to the limbus
- epiphora – watery eye
- enlarged eye(s)
- corneal clouding

Complications
- amblyopia
- myopia which is due to globe enlargement
- reduced vision, even blindness, due to corneal scarring, optic nerve damage

Treatment
Only primary infantile glaucoma is considered here. Treatment of glaucoma associated with other ocular or systemic conditions must be dealt with on an individualized basis. Treatment is primarily surgical, although sometimes additional medical treatment is required by agents used for glaucoma in adults, usually topical β blockers

Surgical
    goniotomy
    trabeculotomy
    trabeculectomy
Medical
    topical ocular hypotensive agents

HYPERTENSIVE RETINOPATHY

The changes in retinal <u>arterioles</u> (there are no true arteries in the retina!) due to systemic hypertension. Unlike any other part of the body these changes can be directly observed. Although hypertensive retinopathy can be graded it is impossible to completely differentiate hypertensive and ageing changes.

Features
- arteriolar attenuation (vasoconstriction) – generalized or focal
- leakage – increased permeability causing haemorrhages and hard exudates

◆ arteriolar sclerosis – thickening of the arteriolar wall with constriction of the arteriovenous crossings (nipping), and copper and silver wiring

Classification (not satisfactory!)
◆ grade 1: generalized arteriolar narrowing and concealment of veins
◆ grade 2: severe generalized attenuation and deflection of veins at crossings
◆ grade 3: arteriolar copper wiring and variation of venous calibre. Haemorrhages, cotton-wool spots and hard exudates
◆ grade 4: all the above plus arteriolar silver wiring and optic disc swelling – papilloedema

Cause
◆ systemic hypertension
◆ malignant hypertension – accelerated severe hypertension causes hypertensive encephalopathy and optic disc swelling, i.e. this last sign is due to raised intracranial pressure rather than the hypertension *per se*

Symptoms
◆ none, unless complicated by late effects of exudation or papilloedema

Complications
◆ vision may be affected if the hypertension is not controlled, e.g. branch retinal vein occlusion

Treatment
◆ treat the hypertension

KERATITIS – BACTERIAL

Bacterial infection of the cornea – AN OPHTHALMIC EMERGENCY

Causes
- large range of gram positive or negative species
- predisposing factors include: corneal abrasion, contact lenses (usually soft), topical steroids, corneal anaesthesia (e.g. previous herpes zoster ophthalmicus)

Symptoms
- red, sticky eye
- pain
- reduced vision
- photophobia

Examination
- conjunctival injection with purulent discharge
- corneal abscess
- may be activity (cells) in anterior chamber

Complications
- severe sight-threatening intraocular infection (endophthalmitis)
- corneal perforation

Treatment
- admit to specialist eye unit – scrape cornea, gram stain and culture
- antibiotics: subconjunctival then intensive drops, e.g. hourly day and night, initially broad spectrum until sensitivities are known
- isolate in cubicle on ward

KERATITIS – MARGINAL

Hypersensitivity reaction affecting the peripheral cornea

Causes
- hypersensitivity to staphylococcal exotoxin

Symptoms
- red eye

◆ discomfort
◆ photophobia

Examination
◆ vision unaffected
◆ conjunctival injection adjacent to area of keratitis
◆ white 'spots' near corneal periphery (limbus) which stain with fluorescein
◆ blepharitis
◆ meibomian cysts
◆ acne rosacea

Complications
◆ occasionally herpes simple keratitis misdiagnosed as marginal keratitis

Treatment
◆ combination of topical steroid and antibiotic gradually tailed off after a few weeks
◆ treatment of underlying lid margin disease (blepharitis)

KERATITIS – VIRAL

Viral infection of the cornea

Causes
◆ herpes simplex type I (commonest)

Symptoms
◆ reduced vision – frequently
◆ unilateral red eye
◆ pain
◆ photophobia

Examination
◆ conjunctival injection
◆ classical dendritic (epithelial) ulcer staining with fluorescein and Rose Bengal
◆ reduced corneal sensation

Complications
- corneal scarring
- may affect deeper corneal layers, e.g. stroma (disciform keratitis)
- corneal perforation
- secondary bacterial infection
- topical steroids contraindicated in dendritic disease
- ulcer may recur

Treatment
- antiviral ointment (e.g. acyclovir) 5x/day initially then gradually taper
- dilate pupil

KERATOCONUS

Corneal dystrophy of unknown aetiology where the cornea progressively adopts a conical rather than spherical shape. Onset usually in late teens

Associations
- none – most cases
- atopy
- Down's syndrome

Symptoms
- progressive blurring of vision due to astigmatism

Examination
- bilateral, often asymmetrical thinning and distortion of inferior and central cornea as it adopts a conical shape
- indentation of lower lid on downgaze (Munson's sign)
- oil drop reflex (stand 2 feet from patient and look at eye through ophthalmoscope)
- fine vertical (Vogt's) lines at apex of cone (seen on slit lamp)

◆ iron (Fleischer) ring around base of cone (seen on slit lamp)

Complications
◆ astigmatism cannot be corrected with spectacles
◆ increased astigmatism leads to contact lens intolerance
◆ central corneal scarring
◆ rapid influx of aqueous into corneal stroma (acute hydrops)

Treatment
◆ gas permeable (sometimes scleral) contact lenses
◆ corneal grafting

LEUKOCORIA

The white pupil, or leukocoria, is one of the most important ophthalmic clinical signs in infants and children. Some of its causes are potentially lethal or may have severe consequences for vision. Usually one eye only is involved.

Causes
consider causes anatomically, working from the front to the back of the eye:
◆ corneal clouding
  – strictly, not leukocoria as in front of the pupil and and partially obscures it
◆ cataract
  – an opacity in the lens, due to many causes including inherited, trauma, eye disease, metabolic disorders such as diabetes, galactosaemia etc.
◆ tumour
  – retinoblastoma is the most important, potentially lethal, cause of leukocoria – and can be bilateral
◆ malformation
  – congenital masses in the vitreous

♦ inflammations
  - toxoplasmosis and toxocariasis
♦ retinopathy of prematurity
  - end-stage when scar tissues fills the globe

Symptoms
♦ usually none as children do not complain of loss of vision of one eye
♦ loss of vision indicates involvement of both eyes

Examination
♦ Ophthalmic
  - white pupil – leukocoria
  - parents may have observed it first on a photograph so look at old photos to determine onset
  - strabismus, which as mentioned elsewhere can be the first sign of a serious ocular or systemic disorder
♦ Systemic
  - every child with leukocoria needs a full paediatric assessment unless there is a good reason for this not be undertaken

Complications
♦ depends on cause

Management
♦ every infant or child with leukocoria needs urgent ophthalmic specialist assessment

Treatment
♦ depends on cause

MALIGNANT MELANOMA

This tumour may originate from many ocular and periocular tissues: ciliary body, iris, conjunctiva and eyelid. However the most frequent site is from the choroid and is the most common intraocular tumour in adult life. Melanoma usually presents between 50 and 80 years of age.

Symptoms
◆ none – usually melanoma is identified as an incidental finding at a routine eye examination (for spectacles)
◆ vision loss
◆ visual field defect if large

Examination
◆ pigmented, raised mass in the choroid in the fundus

Investigation
◆ Ocular
  – B-scan ultrasound examination
  – fluorescein angiography – sometimes
◆ Systematic
  – systematic examination looking for metastases, especially in the liver
  – liver function tests
  – CT, MRI to identify extraocular extension

Treatment
◆ observation – for very small lesion which may grow very slowly clearly an expert's decision
◆ enucleation
◆ radioactive plaques sutured to the exterior of the glove for a few days
◆ laser photocoagulation – only if very small
◆ local resection

MEIBOMIAN CYST

Granuloma of the lipid secreting meibomian glands in the lid (chalazion)

Causes
◆ local dysfunction of meibomian gland lipid
◆ associated with blepharitis

Symptoms
◆ lump on upper/lower lid (commonest lid lump)

Differential diagnosis
◆ stye (infection of eyelash root)
◆ lid tumours, e.g. basal cell carcinoma (rodent ulcer)

Examination
◆ initially presents as an oedematous lid with discrete tender area
◆ resolves into hard lump as surrounding oedema disappears

Complications
◆ unsightly if large
◆ occasionally causes astigmatism by pressing on globe

Treatment
◆ hot compresses
◆ antibiotic drops/ointment
◆ incision and curettage under LA

NYSTAGMUS

Rhythmic oscillation of the eye(s)
   Almost always affects both eyes, but can be asymmetrical, and occasionally is voluntary

Causes
◆ physiological, e.g. calorics, optokinetic, voluntary
◆ sensory deprivation – reduced vision in early life (before 6 years)
◆ CNS causes
   – vestibular – often with a rotatory element
   – cerebellar disease
   – brainstem disorders – many including demyelination

  - vascular lesions and tumours
  - drugs – almost any acting on the CNS – alcohol is the most frequently seen
♦ specific types – there are a number of types such as see-saw, up-beat which provide important clues to the basic pathology
♦ congenital nystagmus – this diagnosis can only be made after all other possibilities have been considered, can be familial

Symptoms
♦ acquired – causes oscillopsia and reduced vision – quite disabling
♦ congenital – reduced vision but no oscillopsia

Examination
♦ examine for a neurological abnormality
♦ examine for an ocular abnormality – which may be subtle and in childhood require electro-physiological testing

Treatment
♦ treat the underlying cause

OPTIC ATROPHY

Atrophy of the optic nerve head (or a part thereof) resulting from damage to nerve fibres at the level of the retina, optic disc or pre-geniculate visual pathways

Causes
♦ retinal
  - retinal artery occlusion
  - retinitis pigmentosa
♦ optic disc
  - vascular: ischaemic optic neuropathy (arteritic and non-arteritic)
  - glaucoma
  - demyelinating disease
  - inflammatory: vasculitis, papillitis

♦ pre-geniculate visual pathways (i.e. optic nerve, chiasm, tract)
  - vascular: ischaemia
  - demyelinating disease
  - compressive (tumour, aneurysm)
  - toxic (drugs) and metabolic, e.g. B12 deficiency, tobacco/alcohol amblyopia, methanol poisoning
♦ congenital/hereditary

Symptoms
♦ those of original cause
♦ loss of vision

Examination
♦ optic disc pallor: whole of disc in optic nerve lesions, may be segmental in vascular disease
♦ characteristic visual field defects depending on site of lesion
♦ afferent pupillary defect may be present

Treatment
♦ treat the fundamental cause
♦ atrophy usually represents irreversible loss of optic nerve fibres so complete restoration of vision unlikely

PAPILLOEDEMA

Swelling of the optic nerve head resulting from raised intra-cranial pressure (ICP)

Causes
♦ obstruction of CSF flow in ventricular system by congenital or acquired lesions such as tumours
♦ obstruction of CSF absorption by arachnoid villi (e.g. blood, protein, inflammatory debris)
♦ obstruction of cerebral venous drainage system
♦ benign intracranial hypertension (BIH)

Symptoms
- those of raised ICP
- transient visual obscurations
- normal vision unless optic atrophy

Examination
- blurring of optic disc margins
- loss of spontaneous venous pulsations
- elevation of optic disc
- hyperaemia and venous engorgement
- haemorrhages and cotton-wool spots
- visual fields full although blind spot enlarged in more advanced cases

Complications
- optic atrophy with visual loss

Treatment
- treat the cause
- in BIH, optic nerve sheath fenestration may prevent loss of vision

Differential diagnosis
- swollen disc due to causes other than raised ICP, e.g. papillitis, vasculitis, optic neuritis, CRVO, ischaemic optic neuropathy, malignant hypertension (these causes usually associated with significant visual loss) and optic nerve head drusen

POSTERIOR VITREOUS DETACHMENT (PVD)

Degeneration of vitreous gel resulting in it separating away from its retinal attachment

Causes
- ageing (commonest)
- myopia
- trauma
- intraocular inflammation

Symptoms
◆ nil
◆ flashes
◆ floaters
◆ may be reduced visual acuity and a field of vision defect if a complication has occurred

Examination
◆ usually nil unless a complication has occurred

Complications
◆ nil
◆ as the posterior vitreous separates it pulls on the retina resulting in
  – retinal tear and subsequent retinal detachment
  – macular hole
  – vitreous haemorrhage (due to avulsion of a retinal vessel)

Treatment
◆ nil unless there is a complication
◆ warn the patient to reattend if symptoms persist or recur

PTOSIS

Drooping of the upper eyelid, may be unilateral or bilateral
  The upper lid normally covers the superior corneal limbus by 1–2 mm

Causes
◆ **Neurogenic**
  – III N palsy
  – Horner's syndrome
◆ **Myogenic**
  – congenital – dystrophic levator palpebrae superioris (LPS), may be associated superior rectus weakness, old photos may be of value for comparison

- myasthenia gravis – variable, fatiguable
- myotonic dystrophy
◆ **Aponeurotic**
  - dehiscence of LPS aponeurosis due to ageing, trauma
◆ **Mechanical**
  - lid lumps
  - inflammation
  - oedema

Symptoms
◆ nil
◆ reduced vision if lid covers visual axis, in children may cause amblyopia (see under **STRABISMUS**) leading to permanent visual loss
◆ cosmetic

Examination
◆ exclude pseudoptosis, i.e. microphthalmic (small) eye, or upper lid retraction/prominent other eye
◆ using clear plastic ruler measure:
  - degree of ptosis (palpebral aperture)
  - LPS function (immobilize frontalis) – normal 15 mm or greater
  - height of upper lid skin crease – a higher crease = aponeurotic defect
◆ check movements of extraocular muscles
◆ assess corneal sensation (ophthalmic division of trigeminal nerve) – use end of a tissue
◆ check Bell's phenomenon – ask patient to squeeze eye very tightly and you forcibly try to open it; as you prise the lids apart the eye should roll upwards and not be exposed = good Bell's
◆ Tensilon test, anti-acetylcholine receptor antibodies (if indicated)

Treatment
◆ treat underlying cause, e.g. myasthenia gravis, lubricants may be required

◆ surgery – type of operation depends on LPS function and degree of ptosis
◆ some do not require treatment

PUPIL RESPONSES – ABNORMAL

Normal
◆ light reflex: direct and consensual
◆ near reflex

Examination
◆ pupil size
◆ asymmetry (which is the abnormal pupil?)
◆ irregularity (previous uveitis)
◆ direct and consensual light reflex
◆ near reflex
◆ for relative afferent pupillary defect (RAPD)

Abnormal
◆ Marcus Gunn (RAPD +ve): reduced optic nerve function (gross retinal disease, e.g. extensive detachment)
◆ Holmes–Adie (tonic pupil, large pupil initially, smaller years later): associated with reduced tendon reflexes, cause obscure, of no significance
◆ Horner's syndrome (oculosympathetic palsy, small pupil more obvious in dim illumination): due to interruption of sympathetic chain
◆ Argyll–Robertson (small pupils, light-near dissociation): syphilis, diabetes
◆ III nerve palsy (dilated pupil, eye abducted, ptosis): posterior communicating artery aneurysm (pupil spared if a medical cause, e.g.diabetes)
◆ drug induced: pilocarpine, cyclopentolate, atropine

Symptoms
◆ usually nil
◆ difficulty in focusing if pupil large

RETINAL ARTERY OCCLUSION

Occlusion of central (CRAO) or branch retinal artery (BRAO)

Cause
◆ atheroma
◆ embolus (usually from carotid bifurcation)
◆ arteritis (especially giant cell arteritis)
◆ raised intraocular pressure

Symptoms
◆ painless, sudden loss of vision in one eye (more severe visual loss cf CRVO)
◆ visual field defect (BRAO)
◆ may have history of amaurosis fugax

Examination
◆ afferent pupillary defect (CRAO)
◆ pale retina with a cherry red spot at the macula (CRAO)
◆ segmentation of blood in the vessels
◆ embolus

Treatment
◆ if within 12 h lower the intraocular pressure (drain aqueous surgically – a specialist procedure) to aid perfusion
◆ after 12 h no immediate eye treatment
◆ systemic evaluation, including an urgent ESR (for giant cell arteritis)
◆ aspirin for amaurosis fugax

Complications
◆ high incidence of other embolic phenomena, e.g. TIA, CVA
◆ optic atrophy (CRAO)
◆ ocular neovascularization

RETINAL DETACHMENT

Separation of the sensory retina from the retinal pigment epithelium. May result in permanent loss of vision if not treated urgently – REFER TO AN EYE UNIT

Causes
◆ retinal tear with influx of fluid between the two layers
◆ associated with posterior vitreous detachment
◆ associated with trauma
◆ commoner in myopes

Symptoms
◆ flashes
◆ floaters (tadpoles, cobwebs)
◆ field loss, opposite direction to detachment
◆ reduced vision, profound if a 'macular off' detachment

Examination
◆ grey, corrugated appearance of retina ballooning forward into the vitreous

Complications
◆ poor recovery of vision due to photoreceptor damage, especially if macula detached prior to surgery
◆ redetachment
◆ glaucoma
◆ blindness if surgery unsuccessful

Treatment
◆ surgical
  – external approach (conventional)
  – internal approach (vitrectomy)

RETINAL VEIN OCCLUSION

Occlusion of central (CRVO) or branch retinal vein (BRVO)

Causes
- atherosclerosis (commonest for CRVO)
- hypertension (commonest for BRVO)
- hyperlipidaemia
- diabetes mellitus
- raised intraocular pressure (CRVO)
- hyperviscosity syndromes
- vessel wall inflammation (retinal vasculitis)

Symptoms
- painless, sudden decrease or distortion in visual acuity in one eye, usually as a result of macular oedema/haemorrhage – can remain undetected for weeks or months (some BRVO are asymptomatic because they do not involve the macula)

Examination
- CRVO
  - swollen optic disc and retina especially macular area
  - marked venous engorgement
  - haemorrhages and cotton wool spots
- BRVO
  - the above signs are confined to one sector of retina

Treatment
- systemic evaluation to determine cause – treat accordingly
- may require laser treatment to prevent ocular complications

Complications
- macular oedema, ocular neovascularization, vitreous haemorrhage, neovascular glaucoma (CRVO)

Conditions

RETINITIS PIGMENTOSA

A heterogeneous group of conditions affecting primarily the retinal rods, and later retinal cones. Relatively infrequent, retinitis pigmentosa (RP) usually commences before adult life, but may start earlier or later. It is untreatable and has progressive course eventually resulting in tunnel vision and blindness.

Cause
◆ inherited by dominant, autosomal recessive and X-linked traits
◆ sporadic

Associations
◆ Ocular
  – cataract frequently develops after many years and which may require surgical treatment
◆ Systemic
  – most RP is an isolated condition, but it can be associated with a large range of conditions involving hearing, motor activity, obesity, polydactyly, cardiomyopathy, etc.

Symptoms
◆ deficient retinal rod function – early:
  – night blindness
  – peripheral visual field loss – tunnel vision
◆ deficient retinal cone function – later:
  – reduced vision

Examination
◆ bone-corpuscular pigmentation alongside the retinal blood vessels

Investigations
◆ symptoms are present before any ophthalmoscopic signs are present, so the diagnosis can only be made by:
  – electroretinography (ERG, discussed elsewhere) which evaluates retinal rod activity
  – visual field analysis

Complications
◆ blindness which occurs at different ages according to the genetic type
◆ cataract

Treatment
◆ none for RP, but treatment of some complications such as cataract can benefit the patient
◆ valuable support can be given to RP sufferers with respect to mobility, rehabilitation, low vision aids etc.

RETINOBLASTOMA

A tumour arising from the retina. Rare but is the most common ocular malignancy of childhood with an incidence of 1 in 20 000 live births. May be present at birth and 90% have presented by 3 years. Familial or sporadic. Familial more likely to be bilateral. Sporadic can be unilateral or bilateral, the latter is considered to be the start of a germinal mutation. Retinoblastoma is a potentialy fatal malignancy which spreads along the optic nerve. Very high cure rate if identified early

Symptoms
◆ none, in most cases – diagnosis is made on signs alone
◆ vision loss if bilateral

Examination

Screening
◆ all babies are routinely screened for the presence of a red reflex within the first 48 h after birth

Specific
◆ the most common presenting signs are as follows:
  – leukocoria (white pupil) – see elsewhere
  – strabismus

- red eye – a very late presenting feature
- orbital inflammation and proptosis

Investigation
- differentiate from other causes of leukocoria and refer to a paediatric ophthalmologist – full paediatric evaluation is necessary after ophthalmic work-up
- ultrasound, CT and MRI scans may all be required

Treatment
- should only be treated in centres specializing in paediatric oncology
  - photocoagulation or cryotherapy for small lesions
  - enucleation – when the eye cannot be saved
  - radiotherapy – often effective

RETINOPATHY OF PREMATURITY

A condition of the retinal blood vessels of babies born prematurely and which is potentially blinding. Most (over 95%) retinopathy of prematurity (ROP) resolves spontaneously without adverse sequelae for the eye and vision.

Causes
- prematurity – both incidence and severity rise with increasing immaturity at birth
- hyperoxia – this relationship is not entirely predictable and ROP can develop without oxygen being administered
- many other factors have been implicated, such as vitamin E deficiency, blood transfusions, cerebral ischaemia and early exposure to light

ROP process
- immature retinal blood vessels proliferate and if resolution does not occur results in the

formation of intraocular scar tissue, distorting the retina and if advanced even occupying the vitreous cavity

Symptoms
◆ none until untreatable problems arise, so see next section

Classification
There is an internationally agreed classification which does not need detailing here

Examination/screening
Because of the non-predictive relationship with illnesses and other risk factors certain babies need to be routinely screened

which babies?
   – ALL under 1500 g birth weight
   – ALL less than 32 weeks gestational age

time of screening examination
   – the time window for treatment is very narrow so:
   – commence 6–7 weeks after birth and screen babies every week or 2 weeks until approximately 37 weeks postmenstrual age

Complications
◆ none for most babies who undergo spontaneous resolution
◆ myopia and other refractive errors as ROP affects the shape of the eye
◆ reduced vision, even blindness

Treatment
◆ cryotherapy or laser therapy delivered at a critical time in the acute phase, lasting only about 1 week, which is usually around 3 weeks before full term

SARCOIDOSIS

A multi-system disorder characterized by the presence of non-caseating granulomas in several affected organs or tissues. A definitive diagnosis can only be made histologically. About one-third of patients with systemic manifestations of sarcoidosis will have ocular involvement. Commoner in 'American' blacks

Clinical features
- ◆ uveitis (intraocular inflammation)
  - – commonest type is retinal vasculitis with panuveitis
    - * retinal periphlebitis (sheathing of veins)
    - * 'cuffing' of retinal veins by lymphocytes
    - * 'candle-wax' exudates (perivenous exudation)
    - * retinal neovascularization
  - – acute/chronic anterior uveitis
- ◆ optic nerve head infiltration by granulomas
- ◆ lacrimal gland infiltration (enlargement)

Associated systemic features
- ◆ abnormal chest X-ray
  - – bilateral hilar lymphadenopathy
  - – pulmonary infiltrate and fibrosis
- ◆ erythema nodosum
- ◆ parotid gland swelling
- ◆ arthralgia
- ◆ lupus pernio (skin lesions)
- ◆ raised serum angiotensin converting enzyme
- ◆ positive Kveim test
- ◆ hypercalcaemia

Ocular complications
- ◆ from the uveitis
  - – cataract
  - – secondary glaucoma
  - – cystoid macular oedema
  - – vitreous haemorrhage

Treatment
◆ corticosteroid
  – topical
  – periocular injection (for sight-threatening complications)
  – systemic ± immunosuppression (for sight-threatening complications)

SCLERITIS

Rare – inflammation of the outer (white) coat of the eye and can be a severe, destructive, sight-threatening disease. Anterior scleritis is commonest but posterior involvement also occurs. Anterior scleritis is sub-divided into diffuse, nodular, and necrotizing.

Causes
◆ majority idiopathic
◆ 25% associated with a connective tissue or vasculitic disease, commonest being rheumatoid arthritis

Symptoms
◆ pain (may be so severe that it wakes the patient at night)
◆ red eye(s)
◆ may be recurrent

Examination
◆ deep red coloration of anterior sclera – may be diffuse or localized
◆ visual acuity may be normal
◆ scleral thinning associated with bluish/black discoloration from underlying uveal tissue

Complications
◆ visual loss
◆ scleral thinning
◆ perforation of the globe
◆ optic disc and macular oedema (posterior scleritis)

Treatment
- ◆ oral non-steroidal anti-inflammatory drugs for mild cases, e.g. flurbiprofen 50–100 mg tds
- ◆ topical steroids as supplementary therapy
- ◆ systemic corticosteroids/pulsed immunosuppression for severe cases

SICKLE CELL RETINOPATHY

Retinopathy associated with certain sickling haemoglobinopathies, e.g. HbSS, HbSC and sickle thalassaemia. The first two are common in people of equatorial African origin while thalassaemia is most frequently seen in those from the Mediterranean area.

Cause

General
- ◆ deformed red cells easily occlude vessels. Occlusion can be precipitated by hypoxia from flying in an airplane or general anaesthetic. Because of the latter, all people of African origin should have a sickle test before being submitted to a general anaesthetic

Ocular
- ◆ occlusion results in neovascularization which is the characteristic response to retinal ischaemia. The characteristic lesion is the 'sea fan' pattern of new vessels and these may bleed, or by fibrosis cause retinal traction and/or detachment

Symptoms
- ◆ none, usual
- ◆ reduced acuity
- ◆ visual field loss
  - – The last two follow a vitreous haemorrhage or damage or detachment of large areas of the retina

Examination

◆ neovascularization in the peripheral retina – very difficult to visualize with the direct ophthalmoscope

◆ vitreous haemorrhage and retinal fibrosis in advanced cases

Treatment

◆ prophylactic – minimize the risk of sickling, by avoiding hypoxic situations

◆ laser photocoagulation or cryotherapy (sometimes) of the ischaemic areas. The approach to treatment is broadly similar to that of other types of ischaemic retinopathy such as diabetic retinopathy.

STRABISMUS

Misalignment of the visual axes

Also commonly known as squint, but by patients also as a 'turn' or 'cast'

Strabismus may be the first sign of a serious neurological or ocular disorder – in other words its significance, as in so many eye conditions, may extend beyond the visual system

Terminology

Two broad categories:

1. paralytic = incomitant
2. non-paralytic = concomitant = comitant

For each of the above, the eyes may be convergent (esotropia) or divergent (exotropia). Vertical deviations can also occur

Consequence of strabismus – amblyopia

Amblyopia is caused by strabismus, refractive errors and any obstacle to the DEVELOPING visual system, such as cataract, ptosis etc.

Amblyopia does not occur after about 6–8 years of age

AMBLYOPIA – reduced vision which persists after the removal of any obstacle to clear vision

Amblyopia treatment

Can only be treated in childhood, therefore it is important to diagnose early

◆ treatment of the underlying cause
  – remove any obstacle to clear vision – cataract, ptosis etc.
  – refractive correction by spectacles or even contact lenses
◆ occlusion therapy – patch the good eye
  – note this is undertaken after management of the underlying cause
  – note the squint does NOT have to be corrected first

Paralytic strabismus (incomitant)

Strabismus due to a cranial nerve palsy (III, IV, or VI)

The usual type of deviation in adults, because of the serious associations, consider a paresis first

Causes
◆ compression, by tumour, aneurysm etc.
◆ infection
◆ muscle disease, e.g. myasthenia gravis
◆ congenital – a diagnosis of exclusion

Symptoms
◆ diplopia when the eyes attempt to move into the direction of the palsied muscle
◆ diplopia which clears when the eyes look away from the palsied muscle, or one eye is covered – binocular
◆ the young child is able to suppress diplopia very quickly and therefore this symptom is not common in childhood
◆ other symptoms dictated by the underlying cause of the strabismus

Examination
- ◆ examine the eye movements in ALL directions – there will be limitation of movement towards the direction of the palsied muscle, sometimes quite subtle
- ◆ consider neurological examination if indicated

Treatment
- ◆ management of the diplopia – (see under **EYE MOVEMENT DISORDERS**)
- ◆ management of the visual consequence of diplopia – AMBLYOPIA (in children only)

Non-paralytic strabismus (comitant)
The commonest strabismus type in children. Infrequent in adults, but may result from a childhood tendency for a squint which somehow does not become manifest until adult life

Unlike paralytic strabismus the ocular movements are full

Causes
- ◆ high refractive errors
- ◆ poor vision of one or both eyes
- ◆ *squint may be the presenting sign of an intraocular tumour such as retinoblastoma*
- ◆ familial
- ◆ premature birth – the incidence of squint in ex-prematures is much higher than normal
- ◆ neurodevelopmental delay – very high incidence
- ◆ unknown – exclude other causes first
- ◆ remember a long-standing squint may be become comitant with time

Examination
- ◆ examine ocular movements in ALL positions
- ◆ perform a cover test, with an interesting target (not a light) at near (33 cm) and distance (6 m)

Treatment

Child
◆ correct any amblyopia first
◆ refractive correction - this is the first part of amblyopia correction, and may also correct the squint itself
◆ surgery

Adult
◆ refractive correction
◆ botulinum toxin
◆ surgery

TOXOPLASMOSIS

Infection by the obligate intracellular parasite, *Toxoplasma gondii* is a well recognized cause of retinochoroiditis. Approximately 30–50% of the adult population will have serological evidence of previous toxoplasma infection.

Modes of transmission
◆ young cats are the definitive hosts and excrete oocytes in their faeces
◆ infection occurs as a result of eating raw/partly cooked meat from other infected animals acting as intermediate hosts
◆ vast majority of ocular infections are recurrences of congenital disease
◆ congenital infection arises when a pregnant woman becomes infected and toxoplasma crosses the placenta to infect the fetus
◆ once maternal immunity has developed, subsequent fetuses will be protected against congenital infection. Likewise, a woman with congenital toxoplasmosis cannot transmit the infection to her children
◆ acquired disease is usually asymptomatic or may take the form of a glandular fever-like illness

◆ AIDS patients are at risk of developing acquired ocular toxoplasmosis as well as reactivation of pre-existing ocular lesions

Symptoms
◆ floaters
◆ reduced visual acuity if the macula or optic disc affected
◆ occasionally red, photophobic eye

Examination
◆ necrotizing retinitis with an associated posterior/panuveitis
◆ active retinitis usually appears as an oval or circular white, fluffy area with overlying vitreous activity
◆ often a reactivation of a previous lesion occurring at the edge of an old scar
◆ inactive lesions take the form of atrophic scars with hyperpigmentation along the borders

Treatment
◆ peripheral retinal lesions require no treatment
◆ systemic treatment is given for vision threatening lesions, i.e. affecting the macula or optic disc
◆ systemic therapy regimens include:
(1) pyrimethamine/sulphadiazine/prednisolone plus folinic acid supplements, (2) clindamycin/sulphadiazine/prednisolone and (3) co-trimoxazole/prednisolone.
◆ measures should be directed at preventing maternal infection during pregnancy
◆ all lesions in AIDS patients require long-term systemic therapy and corticosteroids are not used

Complications
◆ permanent loss of visual acuity as a result of damage to macula or optic disc

TRAUMA

A systematic approach is essential – always work from front to back.

Beware – some of the most serious injuries exhibit few symptoms or signs

The purpose of this section is to alert you to the variety of ophthalmic injuries, and treatment will not be considered.

Surface injuries

Conjunctiva
- only rarely the sole site of injury, however the presence of a subconjunctival haemorrhage (insignificant in itself) can be a clue to a serious underlying problem such as intraocular haemorrhages in non-accidental injury of childhood
- foreign bodies – may lodge on the tarsal surface of the upper lid – examine this area

Cornea
- abrasions – due to blunt injury
- foreign bodies – history is often uninformative: always consider this if there is a red eye, if there is a possibility of an intraocular foreign body X-ray

Chemical injuries
- whatever the chemical – wash out copiously with water: alkalis are particularly damaging

Blunt injuries
caused by squash ball, the gentle application of a fist etc.

Signs
- **hyphaema** – blood in the anterior chamber
- **vitreous haemorrhage** – both of these will cause a black ophthalmoscopic view
- **traumatic mydriasis** – irregular, poorly reacting pupil due to blunt trauma

- ◆ **iridodialysis** – peripheral tear of a section of the iris root
- ◆ **lens** – dislocation or cataract formation
- ◆ **retinal detachment** – particularly likely if there has been a vitreous haemorrhage
- ◆ **orbital damage** – blow-out fracture

Penetrating injuries

A high index of suspicion is essential, for the patient is often unaware of the nature and severity of the injury (also the site of penetration may seal) – external signs can be minimal

If the object penetrating the eye is large, the symptoms and signs are obvious

- ◆ small FBs which can be metallic and of high velocity, typically hammer and chisel injuries (DIY, home mechanics etc.) may pass into the eye with virtually no tissue destruction; thus there are often no, or minimal signs in the eye; however, iron or copper are chemically toxic to the retina so an X-ray is essential to exclude an FB
- ◆ vegetable material (due to gardening or farming injuries) often lead to serious intra-ocular infection

Examination of all injuries

- ◆ take a careful history, ask about hammering and chiselling etc.
- ◆ measure the visual acuity of each eye
  - – unaided
  - – with a pin-hole
- ◆ examine the eyelids for subtle signs of penetration

Do not press on the eye which may be perforated; you may cause the intraocular contents to be extruded!

- ◆ examine the anterior surface of the eye – conjunctiva, cornea and do not forget to evert the upper eyelid to look for foreign bodies etc.

◆ examine the anterior chamber, iris and lens – (measure the intraocular pressure – specialist procedure)
◆ ophthalmoscopy – black view could be due to a hyphaema or vitreous haemorrhage
◆ consider orbit X-ray if there is a *possibility* of an intraocular foreign body or fracture – it is important to have a high index of suspicion in these cases

VERNAL KERATOCONJUNCTIVITIS

Non-infective, chronic, bilateral conjunctival inflammation with exacerbations in spring and summer months. Associated with atopy and commoner in children and young adults

Causes
◆ unknown

Symptoms
◆ itching (may be severe)
◆ watering
◆ mucus discharge
◆ photophobia

Examination
◆ stringy mucus
◆ giant papillae (inflammatory conjunctival overgrowths) in upper tarsus (cobblestone appearance)
◆ follicles (mini-lymphoid aggregates) at superior corneal limbus
◆ white dots (Trantas' dots) at superior corneal limbus
◆ punctate corneal epithelial keratopathy

Complications
◆ corneal ulcer with central plaque preventing healing

Treatment
- topical sodium cromoglycate to stabilise mast cells and prevent histamine release
- topical mucolytic (acetylcysteine)
- topical lubricants
- topical steroids (in severe cases)
- surgical removal of corneal plaque

THE WATERY EYE

Lacrimation (overproduction of tears) and epiphora (defective tear drainage) results in excessive watering. This is a common symptom which although can often be quite distressing does not result in loss of vision

Causes
- overproduction of tears
  - conjunctival/corneal irritation/blepharitis
  - ocular or nasal pain
  - photophobia in infants with congenital glaucoma
- non-apposition of the lower lid to the globe
  - ectropion
  - VII N palsy
- obstruction of the nasolacrimal drainage system
  - infection
    * mucocoele of lacrimal sac (may follow acute dacryocystitis)
    * canaliculitis (actinomyces)
  - infiltration
    * granuloma (Wegener's)
    * tumour
  - congenital
    * failure to canalize lower end of naso-lacrimal duct (infants), may spontaneously canalize up to 1 year after birth
  - trauma

Examination

◆ check conjunctiva and cornea for any aggravating factors

◆ check lids for blepharitis and lower lid malposition

◆ press on lacrimal sac to see if discharge (mucopurulent) from lower lacrimal punctum (mucocoele)

◆ syringe nasolacrimal apparatus with saline via lower lacrimal punctum
  – regurgitation through upper punctum or failure to taste saline indicates blockage

◆ identify site of blockage with dacryocystogram
  – syringe radio-opaque dye via lower lacrimal punctum and X-ray

Treatment

◆ treat appropriate causative pathology

◆ surgery for entropion, VII nerve palsy and obstruction of the nasolacrimal drainage system (dacryocystorhinostomy)

◆ syringe and probe of nasolacrimal duct in infants >1 year

◆ canaliculotomy and debridement for actinomyces

ASSESSMENT

History taking

History of present complaint

◆ symptoms
  - one or both eyes
  - onset
  - duration
◆ vision
  - visual loss – sudden/gradual
  - distortion – central/peripheral
◆ visual field
  - unilateral/bilateral
  - central/ peripheral
◆ colour
◆ floaters
◆ flashes
◆ pain
◆ photophobia
◆ redness
◆ stickiness
◆ watering
◆ FB sensation/irritation
◆ diplopia
  - horizontal
  - vertical
  - binocular
  - monocular

Past ocular history

◆ include refractive (spectacle, contact lens) history

Family history

◆ specifically ask for ocular disease

Past medical history

Drug history

Allergies

General health

Social history
◆ ability to undertake activities of daily living, e.g. read, watch television, see bus numbers, see shop prices, recognize small change etc.
◆ social circumstances
◆ hobbies

If a child include

Obstetric history
◆ pregnancy
◆ birth details
◆ neonatal problems

Developmental history
◆ milestones

Immunisation history

Common symptomatology
Disorders of the visual system manifest in a number of recognized ways, yet patients often have difficulty in explaining visual symptoms

Pain/redness/photophobia/ discharge	= Front of eye
Painless loss of vision	= Back of eye
Misty vision/glare	= Cataract
Distortion of vision/central	= Macula
Distortion of vision/peripheral	= Peripheral retina
Central scotoma	= Macula
Flashes and floaters N.B.	= Vitreous/retina
Chronic open angle glaucoma	= Asymptomatic
Altered colour vision	= Non-localizing

Flashes and floaters
◆ posterior vitreous detachment
◆ retinal tear

- retinal detachment
- vitreous haemorrhage

Transient loss of vision
- unilateral
  - amaurosis fugax
  - giant cell arteritis
- bilateral
  - cerebrovascular insufficiency
  - migraine

Double vision
- binocular (commonest)
  - strabismus
  - concomitant
  - paralytic, e.g. III, IV, VI N palsies
- monocular
  - uniocular
  - cataract

Differential diagnosis of the red eye

Blepharitis
Minimal red eye(s)
Foreign body feeling
No pain
No photophobia
Normal visual acuity
Crusts on lashes
Meibomian cysts
Acne rosacea

Bacterial conjunctivitis
Red eye(s)
Minimal discomfort
No pain
No photophobia
Normal vision
Pus

Viral conjunctivitis
Red eye(s)
Minimal discomfort
No pain
No photophobia
Normal vision
Watery discharge
Associated URTI
Pre-auricular lymphadenopathy

Bacterial keratitis
Red eye
Pain
Photophobia
Reduced vision – usually
Pus
White spot (abscess) on cornea
Predisposing trauma, anaesthetic cornea, contact lens wear

Viral keratitis
Red eye
Pain
Photophobia
Reduced vision – usually
No discharge
Classical dendritic staining pattern of HSV with fluorescein
Reduced corneal sensation
Recurrent

Marginal keratitis
Red eye
Discomfort
Photophobia
No discharge
Normal vision
White spots on peripheral cornea which stain with fluorescein
Blepharitis

Meibomian cysts
Acne rosacea

Acute anterior uveitis
Red eye(s)
Pain
Photophobia
Blurred vision
No discharge
Small pupil
Irregular pupil
Recurrent
Associated HLA-B27 disease

Episcleritis
Red eye(s)
Mild discomfort/ache
No discharge
Normal vision
Recurrent

Scleritis
Red eye(s)
Severe pain
No discharge
Normal vision
Associated auto-immune disease
Recurrent

Angle closure glaucoma
Red eye(s)
Severe pain
Nausea/vomiting
No discharge
Haloes around lights
Reduced vision
Hazy cornea
Semi-dilated pupil
Hypermetropia

Painless loss of vision

Sudden
- ◆ vascular occlusion
  - – venous
  - – arteriolar
- ◆ retinal detachment
- ◆ anterior ischaemic optic neuropathy
- ◆ vitreous haemorrhage
- ◆ age related macular degeneration

Recent
- ◆ cataract
- ◆ age related macular degeneration

Gradual
- ◆ cataract
- ◆ age related macular degeneration
- ◆ open angle glaucoma
- ◆ diabetic maculopathy
- ◆ papilloedema

Painful loss of vision
- ◆ keratitis
- ◆ uveitis
- ◆ angle closure glaucoma
- ◆ scleritis
- ◆ optic neuritis

Visual fields
Representation in space of the extremes of visual sensation

Visual field defects
- ◆ scotoma (isolated, central, centrocaecal): positive – patient sees a grey/black area, negative – patient sees a gap in visual field
- ◆ hemianopia (homonymous, heteronymous; congruous, incongruous)

◆ nature of defect depends on cause and part of visual pathway involved

Important rule: the more posterior the more congruous, i.e. uniocular defect must arise from one eye, and a congruous hemianopia must involve the optic radiation or visual cortex

Causes
◆ multiple and varied
◆ central scotoma: optic nerve lesion (ischaemic, compressive, demyelination), macular lesion
◆ altitudinal: anterior ischaemic optic neuropathy
◆ chronic open angle glaucoma (with increasing field loss)
  – nasal step, temporal wedge
  – superior and inferior arcuate scotomas
  – temporal and central island
  – central island
◆ centrocaecal scotoma: toxic optic neuropathy
◆ heteronymous hemianopia (bitemporal), e.g. pituitary space occupying lesion
◆ homonymous hemianopia: retrochiasmal pathways (vascular, compressive)

Symptoms
◆ often asymptomatic or clumsy behaviour noted by relatives
◆ loss of vision progressive in SOL, sudden in vascular causes

Examination
◆ confrontation to white and red targets (easy, quick and accurate)
◆ perimetry
  – kinetic
    * stimulus of known intensity moved from a non-seeing area to a seeing area
    * Bjerrum screen, Goldmann perimetry (manual)

- static
  * presentation of stimuli of varying intensity in the same position
  * Humphrey field analyser (automated)

Treatment
◆ investigate as indicated by type of defect found
  – treat the cause
◆ some defects may be reversible, e.g. those due to compressive lesions

Fluorescein angiography
A special type of medical photography mainly used to assess the integrity of the retinal and choroidal circulations

Technique
◆ pupils dilated
◆ intravenous injection of 5 ml 10–20% sodium fluorescein
◆ fluorescein absorbs light with a peak wavelength of 480 nm (blue) and emits it with a peak wavelength of 530 nm (yellow/green)
◆ fluorescein carried free in blood (25%) and bound to albumin (75%)
◆ after 20 s the dye appears in the eye and transit through the choroidal then retinal circulation occurs
◆ sequential fundal photographs taken with camera containing appropriate filters allowing the exciting light to be separated from the emitted light

Interpretation
◆ hypofluorescence
  – vascular filling defect
  – masking of normal retinal and choroidal fluorescence by blood or pigment
◆ hyperfluorescence
  – atrophy of the retinal pigment epithelium (RPE)

– breakdown of outer blood–retinal barrier (dye in subretinal space)
– breakdown of inner blood–retinal barrier with leakage from retinal ateries, capillaries or veins
– leakage of fluorescein from retinal or choroidal neovascularization

Uses
◆ assessment of:
  – retinal vasculopathies
    * diabetic retinopathy
      background
      proliferative
    * retinal vascular occlusions
    * retinal vasculitis
  – age-related macular degeneration (disciform type)
  – macular oedema
  – optic disc swelling
  – various other diseases of retina, RPE and choroid

Complications
◆ nausea and vomiting
◆ anaphylactic reactions (may be severe)
◆ yellow/orange skin coloration (instant suntan)
◆ dark urine

Ultrasonography and biometry
Enables the anatomical components of the eye to be studied and measured accurately even if they cannot be visualized. In some instances the ultrasound pattern indicates the pathological nature of a lesion

Method
◆ probe, which oscillates at frequencies of around 10 000 Hz, is placed on the eyelid, or on the surface of the cornea

A scan – measures the length of the eyeball
B scan – gives a cross-sectional image and is useful for investigating pathology in the vitreous, retina and optic nerve – tumours, haemorrhage, retinal detachment, etc.

Uses
◆ ocular biometry – measure the dimensions (usually length) of the eyeball. This is routine before every cataract operation using both A-scan ultrasound and keratometry to measure the sagittal length and corneal curvature, respectively. From these two measurements the refracting power of the eye is determined and the strength of the intraocular lens to be implanted is calculated. This is the most common everyday use of ultrasound.
◆ study interior of the eye – when the media are opaque (i.e. a cataract) ultrasound permits structures within the eye to be studied to determine whether there is any other pathology present, e.g. retinal detachment
◆ study intraocular mass – the nature of a mass within the eye – e.g. look for calcification or dimensions of a tumour.

Electrophysiology
Three electrophysiologial investigations are frequently used in ophthalmology: the electro-retinogram (ERG), electro-oculogram (EOG) and the visually evoked potential (VEP). Each assesses the function of a different part of the visual pathway and all are complementary to the clinical examination.

General indications for use
◆ frequently enables retinal and neurological diseases to be differentiated. Especially useful in conditions with few or no clinical signs

Electroretinogram (ERG)
- ◆ a mass retinal response from the photorecep-tors and other elements
- ◆ does not measure visual acuity *per se*
- ◆ normal in optic nerve and other neurological conditions, e.g. a patient blind with glaucoma will have a normal ERG but abnormal VEP

Use
- ◆ evaluating rod and cone function together or separately
- ◆ abnormal in widespread retinal photoreceptor conditions such as retinitis pigmentosa

Electro-oculogram (EOG)
- ◆ potential between the cornea and retina and reflects activity in the outer retinal layer – the retinal pigment epithelium, but also reflects rod and cone activity. Used less frequently than the ERG
- ◆ does not measure visual acuity *per se*

Use
- ◆ detecting abnormalities of the outer retina
- ◆ abnormal in conditions affecting retinal rods and cones, e.g. retinitis pigmentosa and other inherited disorders

Visually evoked potential (VEP)
- ◆ measures the visual response from the retina along the visual pathway to the cortex. The VEP is, in effect, an anouncement that a visual stimulus has reached the visual cortex
- ◆ requires a functioning retina and an intact visual pathway

Uses
- ◆ test of optic nerve function – one of its major indications
- ◆ demyelinating disease

- optic chiasmal conditions
- diagnosing functional (hysterical) visual loss
- can provide a measure of visual acuity – research tool, not in routine clinical use

Ageing and the visual system

Two aspects of ageing occur concurrently: first, the general ageing and deterioration of tissues and second, the appreciation that there is a predilection for certain conditions to develop at certain ages. Clearly these two processes are not entirely independent. Here the general ageing of tissues will be discussed and not specific conditions such as temporal arteritis which have a tendency to occur after a certain age, in this particular case 60 years.

Eyelids
- dermatochalasis – excessive upper eyelid skin
- entropion
- ectropion

Cornea
- arcus senilis which in the older age group does not indicate an underlying lipid disorder

Intraocular pressure
- this has a tendency to rise with age, some individuals developing ocular hypertension and a few developing true glaucoma, and requiring medication

Iris
- senile miosis, pupil becomes smaller and less mobile with increasing age

Lens
- cataract

Retina
- drusen, white flecks in the deeper retina
- age-related macular degeneration

Visual functions
◆ visual acuity and the ability to determine contrast (i.e. crisp black and white become more grey) deteriorate slightly at great age (>80)

Eye as a clue to metabolic disease
The unique structure of the eye and the ability to visualize tissues which are generally hidden from view provides a fascinating opportunity to visualize physiological and pathological processes. Some of these are listed below simply to provide an indication of the range of conditions.

Eyelids
◆ xanthelasma due to hyperlipidaemia

Conjunctiva
◆ argyrosis – silver staining seen in those exposed to silver either in industry or in medications

Cornea
◆ arcus senilis – lipid deposition, almost universal over the age of 60, but below 50 years may indicate a hyperlipidaemia
◆ crystal formation in cystinosis
◆ brown ring (Kayser–Fleischer) in Wilson's disease – hepatolenticular degeneration, an important diagnostic sign
◆ corneal clouding in mucopolysaccharidoses
◆ corneal deposits from drugs, e.g. amiodarone and chloroquine

Lens
◆ cataracts form in a wide variety of conditions, most important in diabetes mellitus. Much less frequently in hypocalcaemia, galactosaemia, etc.
◆ dislocated lens (ectopia lentis) can occur in Marfan's syndrome, homocystinosis, etc.

Vitreous
◆ asteroid hyalitis in diabetes
◆ amyloid

Retina
◆ diabetic retinopathy
◆ cherry-red spot is seen in certain neurodegenerative conditions, e.g. Tay–Sachs disease
◆ bull's eye lesion at the macula as a manifestation of drug toxicity, notably chloroquine

Optic nerve
◆ optic atrophy in a number of metablic disorders (especially neurodegenerative) and due to drug toxicity, notably anti-TB agents

Orbit
◆ dysthyroid may cause exophthalmos

Genetics in ophthalmology
Genetic abnormalities which affect the eye alone are not lethal and therefore the pool of genetic ophthalmic disorders in the population is quite high. The principles of genetics will not be discussed here, but it will be obvious from the lists below that certain conditions such as retinitis pigmentosa can be inherited by several modes.

Autosomal dominant conditions
One mutant gene is capable of causing the condition. Sex distribution is equal, although penetrance is variable. Dominantly inherited eye conditions include, retinitis pigmentosa, congenital cataract, and systemic conditions such as Marfan's syndrome.

Autosomal recessive conditions
The condition is only expressed if the patient has a double dose of the mutant gene, one from each

parent. Sex distribution is equal. Examples include many inherited retinal problems, albinism, and neurodegenerative disorders such as Tay–Sachs disease.

X-linked recessive conditions
Males are affected, and their daughters are carriers mainly, but not always entirely, unaffected. Examples include retinitis pigmentosa and albinism.

Cytoplasmic or mitochondrial inheritance
As mitochondria are maternally transmitted, this pattern of inheritance superficially resembles an x-linked trait, but more females than would be expected by this latter mode are affected. An example is a form of optic atrophy known as Leber's hereditary optic neuropathy.

Multifactorial inheritance
Many common eye conditions have a familial tendency but do not fall easily into the patterns described above, and appear to be under the influence of both hereditary and environmental influences. These conditions include open angle glaucoma, non-paralytic squint and age-related macular degeneration.

Genetic counselling
Every patient and potential parent has a right to know what information is available on the possible inheritance of any condition. However, it is important that genetic counselling is just that and is not directive. The prejudices or opinions of the clinician must not be imposed. This enables the family to make its own decisions.

Common ophthalmological instruments

Direct ophthalmoscope
- hand-held
- used to visualize retina
- large image size but small field of view
- monocular

Indirect ophthalmoscope
- worn on head
- requires pupil to be dilated
- patient usually lies on couch
- light is shone through a lens (20D) held in front of the eye
- used to visualize retina, particularly peripheral retina
- good for locating retinal tears
- binocular (stereoscopic) view
- large field of view but small image size
- image inverted and back to front
- mirror attachment for teaching
- used in retinal detachment surgery

Retinoscope
- hand-held
- reflex seen in pupil
- part of the refraction routine in testing for spectacles
- also used by optometrists

Slit-lamp microscope
- enables detailed magnified examination of eyelids, conjunctiva, sclera, cornea, anterior chamber, iris, lens, vitreous
- with appropriate lenses will also allow examination of aqueous drainage angle and retina
- used in conjunction with Goldmann applanation tonometer to measure intraocular pressure

Gonioscopy lens
- ◆ placed on cornea
- ◆ used in conjunction with the slit lamp
- ◆ binocular (stereoscopic) view
- ◆ enables visualization of aqueous drainage angle

3-mirror lens
- ◆ placed on cornea
- ◆ used in conjunction with the slit lamp
- ◆ binocular (stereoscopic) view
- ◆ enables visualization of retina including periphery and also aqueous drainage angle
- ◆ good for locating retinal tears

Other lenses
- ◆ 78D, 90D
  - – held just in front of eye
  - – used in conjunction with the slit lamp
  - – binocular (stereoscopic) view
  - – used to visualize retina
  - – pupil need not be dilated
- ◆ various others placed on cornea
  - – for applying argon/Nd YAG laser treatment

Goldmann applanation tonometer
- ◆ measures intraocular pressure (the gold standard)
- ◆ in contact with the cornea (topical fluorescein and anaesthetic used)
- ◆ used in conjunction with the slit lamp

Air puff (Pulsair) tonometer
- ◆ measures intraocular pressure
- ◆ non-contact (does not touch the cornea)
- ◆ used by optometrists

Topics

VISION AND OPTICS

Visual acuity

The ability of the eye to see detail is termed visual acuity. Although distance and near acuities should be checked in all patients, in practice often distance acuity only is measured. Visual acuity should be tested unaided if spectacles are not worn, or wearing spectacles where appropriate (distance spectacles for distance acuity, reading spectacles for near acuity, and bifocals for distance and near acuity), or wearing contact lenses (distance and near acuity).

Distance acuity (Fig. 1) Snellen chart
Each eye is tested separately using a *Snellen* chart. This comprises rows of letters of decreasing size. Under each row of letters is a small number, i.e. 60 (top letter), 36, 24, 18, 12, 9, 6, 5, 4. The lower the number the smaller the letters. Normal distance acuity is the ability to recognize a row of letter(s) at a distance in metres corresponding to the number underneath that row. For standardization purposes a distance of 6 m from the chart has been chosen. Therefore, normal distance acuity means that the row of letters with the number 6 underneath can be read at a distance of 6 m from the chart – written as 6/6.

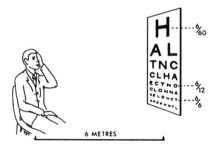

Fig. 1. The Snellen chart.

- Numerator = distance from chart in metres
- Denominator = lowest line of letters seen

Visual acuities less than 6/60 are recorded as follows: 5, 4, 3, 2 or 1/60. Less than 1/60 is recorded as ***counting fingers*** (CF), but if only the movement of the examined hand is seen this is recorded as ***hand movements*** (HM). ***Perception of light*** (PL) is the lowest level of vision recorded, whereafter the patient is completely blind and has ***no perception of light*** (NPL).

The Sheridan and Gardiner test can also be used in patients who cannot read English but are able to match letters. (See Visual acuity testing in children.)

If distance acuity is below normal then the patient should be asked to look through a *pin hole* (or multiple pin holes). This allows only central light rays into the eye and eliminates the blurring of vision due to a refractive error. In general, an improved visual acuity through a pin hole indicates a refractive error is the likely cause of the reduced acuity and not a pathological one; it implies that the patient may require a pair of spectacles or a stronger spectacle lens to give the improved acuity.

Near acuity
This is tested using a standard reading type book held by the patient at a comfortable distance away from them (usually 33 cm). In contrast to distance acuity, both eyes are usually tested together. Normal near acuity is the ability to read a passage of text of size N5 irrespective of whether this is unaided or wearing spectacles or contact lenses.

Refractive error
Blurred vision is most commonly caused by errors of refraction: myopia, hypermetropia, astigmatism. Two-thirds of the refractive power of the eye comes from the cornea and the other one-third from the lens.

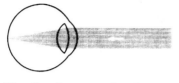

Fig. 2. Emmetropia – image of distant object focused on the retina.

Emmetropia (Fig. 2)
There is no refractive error and light rays from infinity are brought to a focus on the retina. Rays of light from close objects are divergent and are focused on the retina by *accommodation*.

Myopia (shortsighted) (Fig. 3a,b)
Light rays from infinity are brought to a focus in front of the retina either because the eye is longer than normal (axial myopia) or because the converging power of the cornea or lens (index myopia – nuclear sclerotic cataract) is too great.

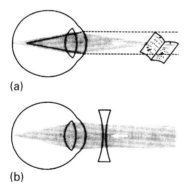

(a)

(b)

Fig. 3. a) Myopia – image of distant object blurred, image of near object focused. b) Correction of myopia – image of distant object focused on retina with concave spectacle/contact lens.

For clear vision the rays of light must be diverged by a concave lens so that they become focused on the retina. For near vision, light rays are focused on the retina with little or no accommodation depending on the degree of myopia and the distance at which the object is held, i.e. myopes can read without spectacles if the text is held close to the eyes. Myopic eyes are prone to retinal tears and subsequent retinal detachment and the optic nerve head (optic disc) is more susceptible to damage by raised intraocular pressure (glaucoma).

Hypermetropia (longsighted) (Fig. 4)
Light rays from infinity are brought to a focus behind the retina either because the eye is shorter than normal or because the converging power of the cornea or lens is too weak. If a cataract is removed and an intraocular lens not implanted the eye is *aphakic* and consequently highly hypermetropic because the converging power of the eye is reduced as it is without a lens. A young hypermetrope may achieve a clear retinal image by accommodating, thus resulting in excellent distance acuity, e.g. 6/4. In moderate/high degrees of hypermetropia or as the person gets older, more accommodative effort is required, especially as the object viewed becomes closer. In this situation a *convex* lens is needed to converge the light rays so that they are focused on the retina.

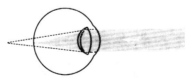

Fig. 4. Low hypermetropia – image of distant object focused on retina by accommodation.

Hypermetropic eyes are more likely to develop acute angle closure glaucoma in later years.

Astigmatism

Occurs when the cornea is no longer spherical and mild degrees are very common. The shape of the cornea is more like a lemon (astigmatism) rather than an orange (no astigmatism). The cornea cannot refract light equally in all meridians, thereby never producing a point of focus on the retina. If one meridian is sharp, the other by definition must be blurred. Correction of astigmatism is with a lens that has power only in one meridian, i.e. *a cylinder*. Astigmatism causes difficulty in seeing both distant and near objects clearly and is frequently combined with myopia or hypermetropia.

Accommodation (Fig. 5)

Physiological mechanism that allows divergent rays of light from close objects (e.g. reading) to be focused on the retina.

In the non-accommodative state the circular ciliary muscle is relaxed, thereby allowing the suspensory ligaments of the lens to remain taut. If accommodation did not take place, divergent rays of light from close objects would be focused behind the retina. To focus the image on the retina (i.e. accommodation) the ciliary muscle contracts and the suspensory ligaments become lax, causing the naturally elastic lens to assume a more globular (convex) shape that has a greater converging

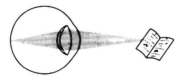

Fig. 5. Accommodation – image of near object focused on retina by accommodation.

power. With age (usually >45 years), the lens gradually hardens and is unable to become as globular as before so that books, newspapers etc. are held further away to reduce the need for accommodation. Thus as close work becomes more difficult, reading spectacles are required – this is known as *presbyopia*.

Spectacles

The power of a spectacle lens is measured in *dioptres* (D). D is equal to the reciprocal of the focal length of the lens, e.g. a lens with a focal length of 25 cm will have a power of 4D.

Convex lenses, i.e. lenses that converge light rays, are indicated by a *plus* sign (+). These lenses are used for hypermetropia, for reading spectacles in presbyopia and various magnifying (low vision) aids. They cause the image of the object to be enlarged.

Concave lenses, i.e. lenses that diverge light rays, are indicated by a *minus* sign (–). These lenses are used for myopia and cause the image of the object to be smaller. The higher (larger) the refractive error of the eye the stronger the lens will need to be to correct it, i.e. more dioptres.

Cylindrical lenses are required to correct astigmatism.

Bifocal lenses are a combination of a lens required for distance vision with another (often smaller) lens at the bottom for reading.

To differentiate between a convex and concave lens hold the patient's spectacles up near your eye and look at a distant object, e.g. edge of a window frame: (a) a convex lens *magnifies*, a concave lens *reduces* the image size; (b) move the spectacle lens a little from side to side; if it is a convex lens the distant object will seem to move in the *opposite* direction to that in which the spectacle lens was moved. The converse is true for concave lenses.

Spectacles give clearer, sharper vision. Not wearing spectacles does not cause any damage to the eye EXCEPT under the age of 8 years, i.e. before the visual system has fully developed; then *permanent reduced* vision may result (*amblyopia*).

Contact lenses
Most contact lenses are worn for non-medical indications (cosmetic) and are used for correcting refractive error, i.e. myopia, hypermetropia, astigmatism. All cosmetic lenses should be worn on a daily basis

Types
◆ rigid gas-permeable (previously called hard)
  – made of polymethylmethacrylate (PMMA)
  – worn on a daily basis
  – smaller than the diameter of the cornea
◆ soft
  – made of hydroxymethylmethacrylate (HEMA)
  – worn on a daily basis
  – include disposable lenses which are replaced frequently
  – more pliable than gas-permeable lenses
  – larger than the diameter of the cornea

Complications
◆ microbial keratitis
  – potentially sight-threatening
    * bacterial
    * acanthamoeba
  – commoner in soft (disposable) lenses, risk increases if worn overnight
◆ corneal hypoxia/oedema/neovascularization
  – increased wearing time
◆ corneal epithelial injury
  – mechanical trauma
  – toxicity of contact lens solutions

- giant papillary conjunctivitis ('cobblestones' under upper lid)
- allergy to contact lens cleaning/soaking solutions

Visual acuity testing in children
Visual acuity develops in childhood and reaches the adult level of 6/6 at around 3–4 years of age. Acuity measurement is very difficult in young children and qualitative assessment is often necessary. The Snellen test, which is used in adults, cannot be used before about 3½ to 4 years of age. Before about 2½ years, and in many older children with learning difficulties, vision cannot be measured directly and qualitative indirect assessments have to be used.

Indirect assessment of vision

History
- parental concern about vision is never ill-founded, but lack of parental concern does not always eliminate a severe defect

Signs
- squint and nystagmus may indicate reduced vision

Direct tests of vision
- following a light or toy, smiling and reaching for an object
- preferential looking-based tests, which are used in specialist clinics. These tests consist of black and white gratings (stripes) which, if seen, generate a looking response from the baby. By presenting narrower stripes visual acuity can be measured

2½ to 3–4 years
- the child holds a card and matches pictures (Kay test) or single letters (Sheridan and

Gardiner) with a card held by the examiner. The most frequently used tests in the preschool child, because Snellen is not possible, but they are less sensitive than the Snellen test and can underestimate the severity of a vision defect

4 years and older
◆ Snellen test; this is the 'gold standard' visual acuity test.

THERAPEUTIC

Ocular pharmacology

Topical preparations
guttae (g.) = drops
oculenta (oc.) = ointment

Common preparations
A number of different drops also come in single dose containers (Minims®)

◆ pupil dilatation and cycloplegia (paralysis of ciliary muscle)
  – g. tropicamide 0.5%, 1.0% (Mydriacyl) duration of action 3 h
  – g. cyclopentolate 0.5%, 1.0% (Mydrilate) duration of action up to 24 h
  – g. phenylephrine 2.5%, 10% duration up to 24 h
  – g. atropine 1% duration of action up to 10 days
◆ for chronic open angle glaucoma
  – beta-blocker
    * g. timolol 0.25%, 0.5% (Timoptol)
    * g. betaxolol 0.5% (Betoptic)
    * g. levobunolol 0.5% (Betagan)
    * g. carteolol 1.0%, 2.0% (Teoptic)
  – sympathetic agonist
    * g. adrenaline 0.5%, 1.0% (Eppy, Simplene)
    * g. dipivefrine 0.1% (Propine)
  – miotic
    * g. pilocarpine 1–4%
  – carbonic anhydrase inhibitor
    * g. dorzolamide 2% (Trusopt)
  – others
    * g. latanoprost 0.005% (Xalatan) – $PGF_2\alpha$ analogue
    * α_2 agonists
◆ antibiotic
  – g. chloramphenicol 0.5% (Chloromycetin)
  – oc. chloramphenicol 1.0% (Chloromycetin)
  – g. fusidic acid 1.0% (Fucithalmic)

- ◆ anti-inflammatory
  - steroid
    - * g. prednisolone 0.5% (Predsol)
    - * g. betamethasone 0.1% (Betnesol)
    - * g. dexamethasone 0.1% (Maxidex)
    - * g. prednisolone 1.0% (Pred forte)
    - * oc. betamethasone 1.0% (Betnesol)
  - steroid/antibiotic
    - * g. Predsol-N (prednisolone 0.5% + neomycin 0.5%)
    - * g. Betnesol-N (betamethasone 0.1% + neomycin 0.5%)
    - * g. Maxitrol (dexamethasone 0.1% + neomycin 0.35%)
  - other
    - * g. sodium cromoglycate 2.0% (Opticrom)
  - antiviral
    - * oc. acyclovir 3.0% (Zovirax)
  - anaesthetic
    - * g. oxybuprocaine 0.4% (Benoxinate)
    - * g. amethocaine 1.0%
  - dyes
    - * g.fluorescein 1.0%, 2.0%
    - * g. Rose Bengal 1.0%
  - lubricants
    - * g. hypromellose 0.3%
    - * oc. simplex (simple eye ointment)

Lasers

<u>L</u>ight <u>A</u>mplification by <u>S</u>timulated <u>E</u>mission of <u>R</u>adiation.

Photocoagulation
- ◆ by argon, krypton or diode laser
  - aim
    - * to create a burn
    - * absorption of light energy by ocular pigments
    - * light energy converted into heat

- indications
  * focal
    ? create adhesion around retinal holes and tears
    ? diabetic retinopathy
◆ panretinal
  - proliferative retinopathies: retinal new vessels due to diabetes or retinal vein occlusion

Photodisruption
◆ by neodyminium-YAG laser
  - aim
    * to disrupt tissues, cells actually explode/ implode
  - indications
    * posterior capsulotomy: to place a hole in the residual posterior lens capsule after cataract surgery
    * peripheral iridectomy: to place a hole in the iris after angle closure glaucoma to prevent further attacks

Photoablation
◆ by excimer laser, just entering clinical practice
  - a controversial topic
  - aim
    * precision corneal ablation – to sculpt cornea
  - indications
    * excision of superficial corneal scars
    * refractive surgery: to help people see better without spectacles, e.g. (myopes)

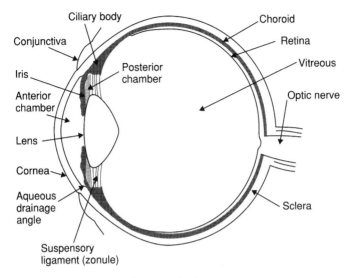

Fig. 1. Cross-section of the eyeball.

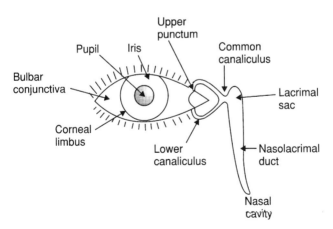

Fig. 2. Anterior view of front of the eye and lacrimal apparatus.

Appendix – useful diagrams

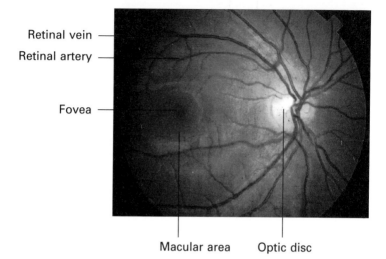

Retinal vein

Retinal artery

Fovea

Macular area   Optic disc

Fig. 3. Ocular fundus.

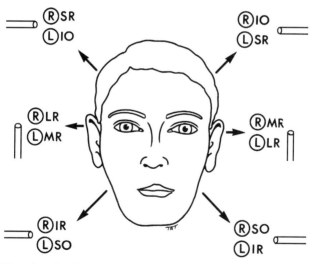

®SR
ⓁIO

®IO
ⓁSR

®LR
ⓁMR

®MR
ⓁLR

®IR
ⓁSO

®SO
ⓁIR

Fig. 4. Ocular movements.

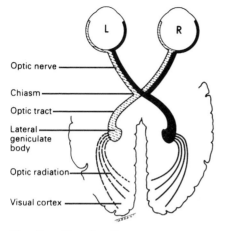

Fig. 5. Visual pathway.

N.B. Page references to illustrations are in bold type.

Accommodation, 91, 93, **93**
Acuity, visual, 8, 89–90
Acute anterior uveitis, 11–12, 75
Ageing, and visual system, 12–13, 14, 31, 47, 82–3
AIDS-related infections, 21 65
Air puff (Pulsair) tonometer, 87
Alkali burns, 13–14
Amaurosis fugax, 32
Amblyopia, 49, 61–4, 95
Angiography, fluorescein, 78–9
Ankylosing spondylitis, 11
Anterior chamber, **103**
Anterior ischaemic optic neuropathy, 14–15
Aphakic eyes, 92
Aqueous
    drainage, 3
    formation, 2–3
    nature and functions, 2
Argyll–Robertson pupil abnormality, 50
Arteriosclerosis, 14
Arteritis, giant cell, 14, 15, 31–2
Arthritis, rheumatoid, 25
Association areas, 7
Astigmatism, 93
Atherosclerosis, 14
Autosomal dominant conditions, 84
Autosomal recessive conditions, 84–5

Bacterial conjunctivitis, 18, 73
Bacterial keratitis, 37–8, 74
Basal cell carcinoma, 15
Bell's phenomenon, 49
Bifocal lenses, 94
Binocular vision, 6, 8–9
Biometry, 79–80

Blepharitis, 15–16, 73
'Blind spot', 5
Blunt injuries, 66–7
Blurred vision, 90
Bowman's membrane, 1
Brain, 8
    visual cortex 6, **105**
BRAO (branch retinal artery occlusion), 51
Brodman's areas, 6, 7
BRVO (branch retinal vein occlusion), 53
Bulbar conjunctiva, **103**
Buphthalmos (ox eye), 35–6
Burns, 13–14

Canal of Schlemm, 3, **103**
Canaliculi, **103**
Cancer, *see* Malignant conditions
Carcinoma, basal cell, 15
'Cast', 61–4
Cataract, 16–18
    formation, 3
    pre-operative procedures, 80
Catheter, venous (Hickman), 22
CF (counting fingers), 90
Chalazion, 43
Chemical burns, 13–14, 66
Chiasm, 5, **105**
Children
    disorders, 35–6, 49, 55–7, 61–4, 95
    visual acuity testing 90, 96–7
Choroid, 42, **103**
    circulation: assessment, 78–9
Ciliary body, **103**
CMV (cytomegalovirus) retinitis, 21–2
Collagen, 4
Colour sense, 8

Index

Concave lenses, 94
Cones, 4, 7, 8, 54, 81
Conjunctiva, **103**
  injuries, 66
  and metabolic disease, 83
Conjunctivitis
  bacterial, 18, 73
  cicatricial, 25
  viral, 19, 74
Contact lenses, 95–6
Contrast sensitivity, 8
Convex lenses, 94
Cornea, **103**
  and age, 82
  components and functions,
    1–2
  dystrophy, 40–1
  foreign body in, 20–1
  injuries, 20–21, 66
  and metabolic disease, 83
  refraction, 1
  see also Epithelium, corneal;
    Keratitis; Keratoconus
Counselling, genetic, 85
Counting fingers (CF), 90
Cranial nerve
  lesions, 30
  nuclei, 8
  palsy, 50, 62
CRAO (central retinal artery
    occlusion), 51
CRVO (central retinal vein
    occlusion), 53
Crystalline lenses, see Lenses,
    crystalline
Cylindrical lenses, 94
Cytomegalovirus (CMV)
    retinitis, 21–2
Cytoplasmic inheritance, 85

Dacryocystorhinostomy, 70
Demyelinating disease, 23–4
Depth, perception of, 9
Descemet's membrane, 2

Diabetic retinopathy, 24–5
Dioptres, 94
Diplopia, 27, 28, 30, 31, 62
Distance acuity, 89–90
Double vision, 73
Drainage surgery, 34
Dry eye, 25–6
Dry mouth (xerostomia), 25
Dyes
  Rose Bengal, 26
  see also Fluorescein
    angiography
Dysthyroid ophthalmopathy,
    26–8

Ectropion, 28
Electro-oculogram (EOG), 81
Electrophysiology, 80–2
Electroretinogram (ERG), 81
Emmetropia, 91, **91**
Endothelium, corneal, 2
Entropion, 28–9
EOG (electro-oculogram), 81
Epiphora, 69
Episcleritis, 29–30, 75
Epithelium, retinal pigment
    (RPE), 4
Epithelium, corneal, 1, 2
  foreign body embedded in,
    20–1
  loss of, 20
ERG (electroretinogram), 81
Eye
  anterior view of front of, **103**
  coordination, 8–9
  maintenance of shape, 2
  power, 1
Eye movement disorders, 30
  nuclear and infranuclear, 30
Eyeball, cross-section, **103**
Eyelids
  and age, 82
  drooping of upper, 48–50
  eversion of lower, 28

inturning, 28–9
margins inflamed, 15–16
and metabolic disease, 83
tumours, 15
see also Meibomian cyst

FBs (foreign bodies), 20–1, 67
Flashes, 72
Floaters, 72
Fluorescein angiography, 78–9
Focusing (accommodation), 91, 93, **93**
Foreign bodies (FBs), 20–1, 67
Form sense, 8
Foscarnet, 22
Fovea, 5, **104**
Foveola, 5

Ganciclovir, 22, 23
Ganglion cells, 4, 5
Genetics, 84–5
Giant cell arteritis, 14, 15, 31–2
Glaucoma, 33–6
acute angle closure, 34–5, 75
chronic open angle, 33
infantile, 35–6
Goldmann applanation tonometer, 86, 87
Gonioscopy lens, 87
Granulomas, 58

Haemoglobinopathies, 60
Haemophilus, 18
Hand movements (HM), 90
Herpes virus, 21, 39
History taking, 71–2
HM (Hand movements), 90
Holmes–Adie pupil abnormality, 50
Horner's syndrome, 50
Hypermetropia (longsightedness), 92, **92**
Hypertensive retinopathy, 36–7

Hypotensives, ocular and systemic, 34

ICP (intracranial pressure), 46
Infection resistance, 2
Inferonasal chiasm, 5
Infranuclear pathways, 8
Inheritance, 84–5
Injuries, 66–8
Instruments, common, 86–7
Internuclear ophthalmoplegia, 24
Intracranial pressure (ICP), 46
Intraocular lens (IOL) implant, 17
Intraocular pressure (IOP), 2, 3
and age, 82
IOL (intraocular lens implant), 17
IOP (intraocular pressure), 3
Iris, **103**
and age, 82
inflamed, 11
Ischaemic optic neuropathy, anterior, 14–15

Kay test, 96
Keratitis
bacterial, 37–8, 74
disciform, 40
marginal, 38–9, 74–5
viral, 39–40
Keratoconjunctivitis, 19, 25
vernal, 68–9
Keratoconus, 40–1

Lacrimal apparatus and lacrimation, 69, **103**
Lasers, 100–1
Lateral geniculate nucleus (LGN), 6, **105**
Lenses
instrumental, 87
spectacle, 94

Index

Lenses, crystalline, **103**
  and age, 82
  implants, 17–18
  and metabolic disease, 83
  nature and functions, 3
  opacification, *see* Cataract
Lesions
  infranuclear, 8
  medial longitudinal
     fasciculus, 24
  optic nerves, 5, 7
Leukocoria, 41–2, 55, 56
LGN (lateral geniculate
  nucleus), 6, **105**
Light sense, 7
Limbus, corneal, **103**
Longsightedness
  (hpermetropia), 92, **92**

Macular area, 4–5, 7, **104**
  age-related degeneration,
    12–13
Maculopathy, 24
Malignant conditions, 15, 42–3,
  55–6
Marcus Gunn pupil
  abnormality, 50
Marginal keratitis, 38–9, 74–5
Measuring and studying
  components of eye, 79–80
Medial longitudinal fasciculus,
  lesions, 24
Meibomian cyst, 43–4
Melanoma, malignant, 42–3
Metabolic disease, eyes as clue
  to, 83–4
Meyer's loop, 6
Microscope, slit lamp 86
Mitochondrial inheritance, 85
MS (multiple sclerosis), 23
Muscle disease, 30
Myopia (shortsightedness), 91,
  91

Nasolacrimal duct, **103**
Near acuity, 90
Neuritis, optic, 23
NPL (no perception of light),
  90
Nystagmus, 44–5

Ocular movements, **104**
Ophthalmopathy, dysthyroid,
  26–8
Ophthalmoplegia, internuclear,
  24
Ophthalmoscopes, direct and
  indirect, 86
Optic atrophy, 45–6
Optic chiasm, 5, **105**
Optic disc, 5, **104**
  cupping of, 33
Optic nerve, 5, **103**
  fibres, 5, 6, 7
  and metabolic disease, 84
Optic nerve head
  arteries supplying, 14
  atrophy, 45–6
  swelling, 46–7
Optic neuritis, 23
Optic radiations, 6, **105**
Optic tract, 6, **105**
Orbit
  changes, 26
  and metabolic disease, 84
Oscillation of eye, 44–5

Papilloedema, 46–7
Paralytic strabismus
  (incomitant), 62
Parastriate and peristriate
  areas, 7
Penetrating injuries, 67
Perception of light (PL), 90
Pharmacological preparations,
  99–100
Photoablation, 101
Photocoagulation, 100–1

Photodisruption, 101
Photopic vision, 7
Photoreceptors, 4
Pin-hole sight testing, 90–1
PL/NPL (perception/no
    perception of light), 90
Posterior vitreous detachment
    (PVD), 47–8
Presbyopia, 94
Pseudoptosis, 49
Ptosis, 48–50
Pulsair (air puff) tonometer,
    87
Punctum, upper, **103**
Pupil
    reflex, 6
    responses, 50–1
    white, 41–2
PVD (Posterior vitreous
    detachment), 47–8

RAO (retinal artery occlusion),
    51
Red eye, differential diagnosis,
    73–5
Refraction, 2
    refractive error, 90–3
Retina, **103**
    and age, 82
    arterioles, 36
    artery, **105**
    artery occlusion (RAO), 51
    circulation: assessment, 78–9
    composition, 4–5
    detachment, 52
    function, 1
    and metabolic disease, 84
    microcirculation disease,
        24–5
    nasal, 5, 6, 7
    substances toxic to, 67
    temporal, 5, 6
    vein, 53, **105**
    see also Cones; Rods

Retinitis
    cytomegalovirus (CMV),
        21–2
    pigmentosa (RP), 54–5, 84
Retinoblastoma, 55–6
Retinochoroiditis, 64
Retinopathy
    diabetic, 24–5
    of prematurity (ROP),
        56–7
    sickle cell, 60–1
Retinoscope, 86
Retinotherapy, hypertensive,
    36–7
Rhodopsin, 8
Rodent ulcers, 15
Rods, 4, 7, 54, 81
ROP (Retinopathy of
    prematurity), 56–7
RP (retinitis pigmentosa), 54–5,
    84
RPE (retinal pigment
    epithelium), 4

Sarcoidosis, 58–9
Schirmer test, decreased, 26
Sclera, **103**
    inflammation of tissue
        covering, 29–30
    nature and functions, 2
Scleritis, 59–60, 75
Scotopic vision, 7
Sheridan–Gardiner test, 90
Shortsightedness (myopia), 91,
    91
Sickle cell retinopathy, 60–1
Sjögren's syndrome, 25
Slit lamp examination, 11
Snellen chart, 89–90, **89**, 97
Sodium fluorescein, 78–9
Spectacles, 94
Squint, 61
Staphylococcus, 15, 18, 38

Strabismus, 61–4
  non-paralytic (comitant),
    63–4
  paralytic (incomitant), 62–3
Streptococcus, 18
Stroma, 2
  foreign body embedded in,
    20–1
Supranuclear disorders, 31
Supranuclear pathways, 8
Surface injuries, 66
Suspensory ligament, **103**
Symptomatology, common,
  72–3

Tear film abnormalities, 25–6
Tear secretion, decreased, 25
Thalassaemia, 60
Thyroid gland dysfunction, 26
Tonometers, 86, 87
Toxoplasmosis, 64–5
Transduction, 1
Transparency, 3
Trauma, 66–8
  see also Lesions
'Turn', 61–4

Uhthoff's phenomenon, 23
Ultrasonography, 79–80
Uveitis, 58
  acute anterior, 11–12, 75

Vasculitis, systemic, 31–2
VEP (visually evoked
    potential), 81
Vernal keratoconjunctivitis,
    68
Viral conjunctivitis, 19, 74
Vision loss
  painless and painful, 76
  transient, 73
  see also Glaucoma
Visual acuity testing, 8, 89–90
  children, 90, 96–7
Visual association areas, 7
Visual cortex, 6, **105**
Visual field defects, 76–8
  central field, 12
  'pie-in-the-sky', 6
Visual functions, and age, 83
Visual information, integration,
    8–9
Visual pathway, 1, 6, **105**
  anterior, 1
  fibre arrangement, 7
  posterior, 1
Visual processing, 7–8
Visual system
  components, 1
  inversion, 7
  requirements, 1
Visually evoked potential
    (VEP), 81

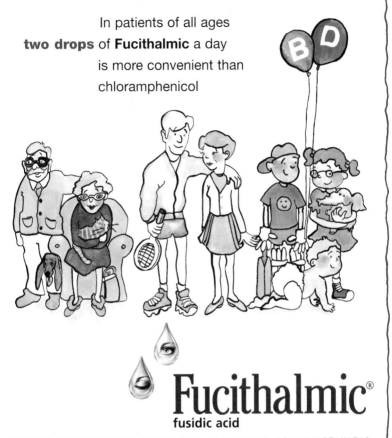

In patients of all ages
two drops of **Fucithalmic** a day
is more convenient than
chloramphenicol

Fucithalmic®
fusidic acid

CHOOSE FUCITHALMIC FIRST, FOR BACTERIAL CONJUNCTIVITIS

2083